the

About.com guide to

HAVING A BABY

Important Information, Advice, and Support for Your Pregnancy

Robin Elise Weiss, LCCE

Adams Media
Avon, Massachusetts

About **About**.com

About.com is a powerful network of 500 Guides—smart, passionate, accomplished people who are experts in their fields. About .com Guides live and work in more than twenty countries and celebrate their interests in thousands of topics. They have written books, appeared on national television programs, and won many awards in their fields. Guides are selected for their ability to provide the most interesting information for users, and for their passion for their subject and the Web. The selection process is rigorous—only 15 percent of those who apply actually become Guides. The following are some of the most important criteria by which they are chosen:

- High level of knowledge/passion for their topic
- Appropriate credentials
- Keen understanding of the Web experience
- Commitment to creating informative, actionable features

Each month more than 48 million people visit About.com. Whether you need home repair and decorating ideas, recipes, movie trailers, or car buying tips, About.com Guides can offer practical advice and solutions for everyday life. Wherever you land on About.com, you'll always find content that is relevant to your interests. If you're looking for "how to" advice on refinishing your deck, About.com will also show you the tools you need to get the job done. No matter where you are on About.com, or how you got there, you'll always find exactly what you're looking for!

About Your Guide

 ROBIN ELISE WEISS (BA, ICCE-CPE, CD[DONA], LCCE, FACCE) is a childbirth and postpartum educator, doula, doula trainer, and proud mother of seven children. She has two passions: pregnancy and writing. A fusion of the two allows her to share her knowledge with others in the classroom, through her books, and on the Web. Since 1989, Robin has attended hundreds of births in a variety of settings, and educated couples about pregnancy and birth. She is the author of several books, including *The Everything® Pregnancy Fitness Book, The Everything® Getting Pregnant Book, and The Everything® Mother's First Year Book.*

Acknowledgments

This book is dedicated to my daughter, Ada. Being number seven has its benefits.

I would like to thank the strong women in my life for the support and love they have given me: Teri Shilling, Pat Predmore, Kim Goldman, Eve Hiatt, Paula Pepperstone, Elizabeth Pedley, Courtney Shaheen, Marci Yesowitch Hopkins, Krista Beck Gallagher, Angela Young, Ashley Benz, and Bekki Williams.

To babies Sam and Charlie for a tough lesson about life: It is always precious, no matter how brief.

To my hand-holding, supportive agent Barb Doyen and editor Katie McDonough.

To my strong, wonderful, and wise children: Hilary, Benjamin, Isaac, Lilah, Owen, Clara, and Ada.

And to the love of my life, Kevin, for supporting my passion for helping women and their families welcome babies into the world, for holding my hand as I labored, and for cradling our babies next to your heart and mind.

"We have a secret in our culture, and it's not that birth is painful. It's that women are strong."

—LAURA STAVOE HARM

ABOUT.COM

CEO & President
Scott Meyer

COO
Andrew Pancer

SVP Content
Michael Daecher

VP Marketing
Lisa Abourezk

Director, About Operations
Chris Murphy

Senior Web Designer
Jason Napolitano

ADAMS MEDIA

Editorial

Publishing Director
Gary M. Krebs

Associate Managing Editor
Laura M. Daly

Development Editor
Katie McDonough

Marketing

Director of Marketing
Karen Cooper

Assistant Art Director
Frank Rivera

Production

Director of Manufacturing
Susan Beale

Associate Director of Production
Michelle Roy Kelly

Senior Book Designer
Colleen Cunningham

Published by Adams Media, an F+W Publications Company
57 Littlefield Street
Avon, MA 02322
www.adamsmedia.com

ISBN 10: 1-59869-095-7
ISBN 13: 978-1-59869-095-8

Printed in China.

J I H G F E D C B A

Library of Congress Cataloging-in-Publication Data
is available from the publisher.

This publication is designed to provide accurate and authoritative information with regard to the subject matter covered. It is sold with the understanding that the publisher is not engaged in rendering legal, accounting, or other professional advice. If legal advice or other expert assistance is required, the services of a competent professional person should be sought.
—From a *Declaration of Principles* jointly adopted by a Committee of the American Bar Association and a Committee of Publishers and Associations

Many of the designations used by manufacturers and sellers to distinguish their product are claimed as trademarks. Where those designations appear in this book and Adams Media was aware of a trademark claim, the designations have been printed with initial capital letters.

This book is available at quantity discounts for bulk purchases. For information, please call 1-800-872-5627.

How to Use This Book

Each About.com book is written by an About.com Guide—an expert with experiential knowledge of his or her subject. While the book can stand on its own as a helpful resource, it can also be coupled with the corresponding About.com site for even more tips, tools, and advice to help you learn even more about a particular subject. Each book will not only refer you back to About .com, but it will also direct you to other useful Internet locations and print resources.

All About.com books include a special section at the end of each chapter called Get Linked. Here you'll find a few links back to the About.com site for even more great information on the topics discussed in that chapter. Depending on the topic, these could be links to such resources as photos, sheet music, quizzes, recipes, or product reviews.

About.com books also include four types of sidebars:

- **Ask Your Guide:** Detailed information in a question-and-answer format
- **Tools You Need:** Advice about researching, purchasing, and using a variety of tools for your projects
- **Elsewhere on the Web:** References to other useful Internet locations
- **What's Hot:** All you need to know about the hottest trends and tips out there

Each About.com book will take you on a personal tour of a certain topic, give you reliable advice, and leave you with the knowledge you need to achieve your goals.

CONTENTS

CONTENTS . . . *continued*

Introduction from Your Guide

Unless you've been living under a rock, you've probably gotten the drift from society that pregnancy and birth are torturous events that one must suffer through before having a baby. The good news is that this is not true. No matter how you choose to give birth, you can have a joyous pregnancy, birth, and postpartum experience.

Learning how to ignore the negative ninny who only wants to share her horror story is only one way to help fight the negative flow of information that seems to come pouring in with the announcement of your pregnancy. You need to be able to surround yourself with people who have a positive, proactive, and reasonable outlook on pregnancy and parenting. You'll soon learn that you can stand up for yourself without ticking off friends and neighbors.

Having faith in your body is not enough to guide the process of pregnancy smoothly through these potentially negative waters. You must also have faith in those you have chosen to help you—from your husband, friends, and family to your practitioner and other health-care professionals. This birth team must share your belief in birth as a positive and empowering experience.

By using the information that you have readily at your fingertips in the form of books, Web sites, and classes, you can learn to take an important role in your health care as a partner. I intend to show you how to build confidence in yourself, your body, and your baby to prepare for the miracle of birth and the joy and excitement of postpartum. By navigating the waters of pregnancy with self-assuredness and knowledge, you can take the helm in this empowering experience of birth, safely and comfortably.

Starting off with such a positive experience will help equip you with the tools you need at 3 A.M., when your reserves are low and you have to get up to feed the baby. These powerful lessons will also get you through hormonal highs and lows with the knowledge of what is normal and what needs help. The key to this positive experience is how you are treated, both during your pregnancy and after, and how you are allowed to make decisions for your family. By exploring your options and choosing what is right for your family, you experience personal growth. This allows you to make the hard decisions that parenting often necessitates.

In the end it is not important whether you gave birth vaginally or without medications, by cesarean or with an epidural. It doesn't matter whether you had a whole range of high-tech tests during your pregnancy or opted out of every single one. The important thing is to make the best choices possible, based on the information available to you at the time. You want to be respectfully listened to and cared for during this sensitive time in your life.

To achieve this, you must learn and grow in the ways of pregnancy. You must educate yourself on what your choices really are. After all, if you only know one thing, what options do you really have? Take that first empowering step toward achieving an amazing birth and turn the page. This book, in conjunction with my About. com site, will guide you along the path to motherhood.

Chapter 1

Getting Pregnant

Preparing for Pregnancy

Do you remember sitting around daydreaming as a child about your family-to-be? Or maybe you and your honey spent some long romantic nights talking about your future children. Maybe you picked out some names and argued over which features your child would get from each of you. These are all fond memories and good experiences, but the reality of having a child is a different story.

A lot goes into planning for pregnancy these days. Men and women are both more acutely aware of the mental and emotional energy they need to be ready for parenthood. The question is, are you ready?

Get your body ready before getting pregnant. One of the best ways to help ensure a healthy pregnancy is to actively prepare to get pregnant before conceiving. This usually entails taking a series of steps leading to an overall healthy lifestyle.

Most families start by eliminating social drugs like alcohol and tobacco from their lives. This is not easy for everyone, but there

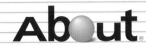

▶ American Legacy's Great Start Program (www.americanlegacy.org/greatstart/html/home.html) is an awesome smoking cessation program specifically designed for mothers-to-be and those trying to get pregnant. Not only does the site explain the advantages to you and your baby of not smoking, but it also provides the support you need to quit for good.

are some great programs available to help you in your decision to have a healthy pregnancy. For best results, get your spouse to join you in quitting.

Cigarette smoke can greatly affect pregnancy. Smoking decreases the amount of oxygen available to your baby via the placenta and makes you more prone to placental problems, miscarriage, stillbirth, and even a premature baby. Quitting before you get pregnant is the ideal. Several mothers-to-be on my About.com forums have said that their first symptom of pregnancy was that cigarettes started to seem nasty to them. Even if you are already pregnant, quitting now drastically reduces your baby's likelihood of developing serious problems from smoking.

Alcohol is another big no-no in pregnancy. There is no safe level of alcohol while you're expecting. In fact, even a single drink at just the wrong time could have disastrous effects on your baby. Alcohol in pregnancy is known to increase the risk of miscarriage. Fetal alcohol syndrome (FAS) and fetal alcohol effects (FAE) both describe certain symptoms displayed by babies (and endured throughout their lives) whose mothers who drank in pregnancy. Do yourself a favor and quit drinking before trying to get pregnant.

Ensuring your body is healthy also includes eating well. Simply being aware of what you eat can be very beneficial. One of the easiest things to do to improve your health is to add more fruits and vegetables to your diet.

Exercise is also a must for a healthy body. Did you know that exercising during pregnancy could help shorten labor and make your recovery go more quickly? To get a jump-start, you need to do this before you get pregnant. Something simple like walking or swimming is all that is needed to have a healthy body, though you also have many other choices, including aerobics, Pilates, or yoga.

A physical checkup is important, too. To figure out and address any potential risk factors, a visit to your midwife or doctor is in order before you get pregnant. For example, if you have high blood pressure, you should get this under control in order to help prevent any of the negative side effects associated with high blood pressure in pregnancy. You should also have a pelvic and a breast exam.

You and your practitioner will decide how you need to prepare to get pregnant. This should include blood work to measure blood sugar and screen for anemia, thyroid disease, and immunities to rubella, as well as other tests as needed. You should also get information about coming off birth control, if applicable. If you have had a baby before, you may also want to discuss health concerns that may have cropped up during your last pregnancy.

In a perfect world, you would be at your ideal weight. Since being over- or underweight can lead to fertility and pregnancy complications, the sooner you reach an ideal weight, the better off you are. Many moms say that switching to a healthier diet and adding exercise helps them find the right balance no matter where they were before getting pregnant.

To sum up, your prepregnancy health checklist should include the following:

- Cutting out risky behaviors, such as smoking and drinking
- Eating a healthy diet with many fruits and vegetables
- Starting or continuing an exercise program
- Visiting your health-care practitioner for breast and pelvic exams, blood work, and discussion of birth control
- Taking prenatal vitamins
- Maintaining weight in normal range

Is this your first baby? If so, you have more things to think about than someone who has already made the transition to

ASK YOUR GUIDE

Is it true that caffeine has the potential to delay conception?

▶ Yes. Some studies also suggest that a higher intake of caffeine leads to an increase in risk to your baby, including premature birth and low birth weight. One study even showed a link between miscarriage and caffeine use. Most problems with caffeine are associated with drinks like coffee and tea. For example, an ounce of dark chocolate has about 20 mg of caffeine, while an eight-ounce cup of coffee can have over 200 mg.

parenthood. Here are some of the things to consider before conceiving:

- ○ Have you had a preconception checkup?
- ○ Have you checked your medical insurance to see what it covers?
- ○ Have you familiarized yourself with your employers' maternity and paternity leave policies?
- ○ Have you discussed genetic testing?
- ○ Have you discussed parenting styles and philosophies?

These conversation-starters are great ways to get comfortable with the subject of becoming parents. Some couples find it easier to sit down and have fixed discussions on the topic, while others prefer to talk about things as they come up. The style of communication that works for you is what you should do.

One woman wrote me to share that she and her husband wrote out answers to their questions and compared notes. This way, they could communicate their thoughts clearly and then discuss each point to find a happy medium. "Waiting for the right time" is a phrase I often hear from people trying to decide when to have a baby. This might mean the right job, the right house, or the right time in a relationship. While it's good to be prepared, if you were to wait for the "perfect" time, you might never have a baby.

While half of all pregnancies are still unplanned, a planned pregnancy is the best option. At the same time, waiting for the perfect time might mean missing other times that are near optimal. Try to balance perfection with reality when deciding to have a baby.

Are you ready for another baby?   Only you and your husband can answer that important question. You might already have talked about it in general terms, but now it is time to discuss the specifics.

▶ Before visiting your practitioner, you will want to gather a list of questions you have about pregnancy and planning to get pregnant. You should ask about any current or chronic health conditions that either you or your husband suffers from. You can include any questions you have about genetic issues. Ask who you can talk to about your physical, mental, and emotional concerns about pregnancy and parenting. Many practices provide such counseling services or can refer you to someone who can help.

Before your first baby, maybe you wanted two kids, but now you're not sure you're ready for a second, now or ever. Keeping a dialogue going is the best way to stay in sync with each other.

There are considerations that come with having another baby, some physical and some decidedly practical or emotional. One question moms ask me before having another baby is whether they will be able to love another child as they do the first. The answer is a decided yes! Here are a few questions you may want to discuss before getting pregnant again:

- ○ Are we physically ready for another baby?
- ○ Do we have room in our home?
- ○ Do we have maternity coverage in our medical insurance?
- ○ Are we emotionally ready to add another child to our life?
- ○ Have we dealt with any issues left over from our previous pregnancy or birth?
- ○ Is there anything physically stopping us?
- ○ Is our child ready to become a sibling?

Even if you have the pregnancy and birth thing down, having another baby means new challenges—like taking care of a child while you're pregnant. If you're really tired and need a nap, you can't simply come home and lie down. You need to convince your first child that a nap is a good idea.

This aside, second pregnancies are different from the first. For one, you know the basics (though you will come to realize that no two pregnancies are identical). If you spent all of your first pregnancy vomiting and are really dreading that happening this go-round, you might be pleasantly surprised to find that you are not sick that often—if at all. (Of course, the opposite is also possible!)

I found that with my second pregnancy, my body started looking and feeling pregnant much sooner. It was like my uterus was

TOOLS YOU NEED

▶ If you have not already started taking a prenatal vitamin or a multivitamin with at least 400 micrograms of folic acid, one will be prescribed for you. For most women, there is little difference between over-the-counter and prescription vitamins. Some health insurance plans do cover the prescription variety. Be sure to talk to your practitioner about your various choices of vitamins.

I've heard that bathing in hot water while pregnant can be detrimental. Is this true?

▶ Despite the old wives' tales, bathing in pregnancy is completely safe. Please bathe! Just remember that an extremely hot bath, shower, sauna, or hot tub can raise your core temperature, which could affect the baby's development. I generally tell mothers-to-be to avoid any water hotter than about 100 °F, though some suggest lower. If you are sweating or feeling uncomfortably hot or dizzy, get out of the tub. For extra security, keep a bath thermometer nearby when you bathe.

thinking, "Oh yes, I know how to do this!" Other moms write to say that they also get this sense of showing sooner. Along with showing sooner, if you've had a previous baby, you're more likely to know what a baby moving feels like and to identify it sooner than a first-time mom would.

Conception Basics

You might be surprised at how much there is to learn before you get pregnant. You may know the basics, or perhaps you just need a refresher course. Think back to sixth-grade anatomy classes—boys and girls have different parts.

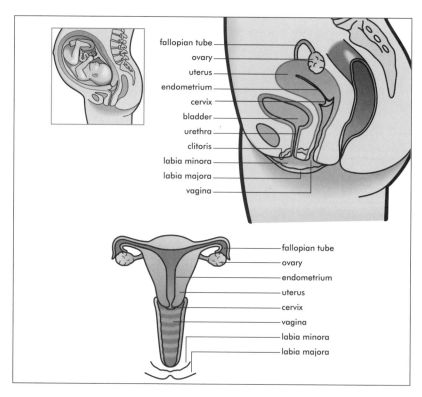

▲ The female reproductive system

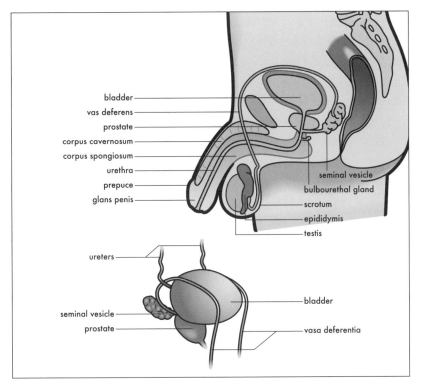

bladder
vas deferens
prostate
corpus cavernosum
corpus spongiosum
urethra
prepuce
glans penis

seminal vesicle
bulbourethal gland
scrotum
epididymis
testis

ureters

seminal vesicle
prostate

bladder

vasa deferentia

▲ The male reproductive system

Here's the rundown. In a woman's ovaries, an egg or ovum is produced about every twenty-eight days. This ovum travels from the ovary to the fallopian tube. In the fallopian tube, it potentially meets sperm that has entered the woman's uterus through her cervix. If the sperm and the egg join, the result is a blastocyst, which continues down the tube to implant into the endometrial lining of the uterus.

It's really all about the timing. You can have sex, but if there isn't an egg or sperm or a uterine lining, there won't be a pregnancy. The key to getting pregnant is to have sex around the time of ovulation.

ASK YOUR GUIDE

Is there one position for intercourse that works better for getting pregnant?

▶ Basically any position that gets the semen to the cervix, where it needs to be, does the job. That said, there are some sexual positions that do not work well when it comes to getting pregnant. Standing and woman-on-top positions can be less effective. That old standby, the missionary position, works well for most couples. You can even try to boost this position with a pillow under your hips.

Ovulation occurs at a certain point in the menstrual cycle. Typically, ovulation occurs fourteen days before the start of your period. Day one of your menstrual cycle is the first day of bleeding. So, if your cycle is twenty-eight days long, you most likely ovulate around day fourteen. If your cycle is thirty days long, you most likely ovulate around day sixteen.

Not everyone has predictable cycles or ovulation. Some women who write to me say that their cycles are all messed up, with no predictable pattern. Generally, we talk about charting their cycles on paper or on the computer. It is only then that they write back to say they do see a pattern—just not a monthly one.

If you have questions about when you ovulate or your cycle, be sure to check in with your midwife or doctor. Sometimes determining when you ovulate is harder to do for a variety of reasons. This does not necessarily mean that you have a fertility problem. Your practitioner will be more than willing to help you figure out your cycle and achieve your pregnancy.

Am I Pregnant?

If you have been trying to get pregnant, you may be really anxious to find out if all of your planning worked. You may be waiting for your next period, or you might be wondering what's up with your body as you experience new sensations or symptoms. Here are some of the most common pregnancy symptoms:

- Missed or abnormal period
- Sensitive breasts
- Fatigue
- Nausea and/or vomiting
- Increased urination
- Feeling of bloating or fullness in the lower abdomen

▶ Fertility monitors are handy items to have around. There are a couple of different kinds available. The MaybeMOM™ (www.maybemom.com) is a small lipstick-sized device that uses saliva. The ClearPlan Easy Fertility Monitor (www .clearplan.com), on the other hand, uses your urine to test for certain hormones that indicate ovulation is near.

Any of these symptoms may indicate pregnancy. Taking a pregnancy test is the easiest way to find out if you are pregnant. Most home pregnancy tests can be taken as early as the first day after your missed period.

Whole shelves of pregnancy tests are available at nearly any store. Do not get overwhelmed by the sheer number of options available. Simply pick a test in your price range and take it. Yes, there are some basic differences, but for the average woman, nearly any test will do. The most expensive test is not always the most sensitive.

Pregnancy tests are pretty accurate. If the stick turns blue, shows two lines, or does whatever it's supposed to do to show you a positive sign, chances are very good that you are pregnant! If the test is negative and your period is late, the instructions will usually tell you to wait a few days and repeat the test. This is because the pregnancy hormone, hCG, doubles nearly every forty-eight hours. If you haven't gotten your period or a positive pregnancy test within a week, make an appointment to see your practitioner.

After your positive pregnancy test, the next step is to make an appointment with your midwife or doctor. More and more women are writing me to say that they are being put off for this first appointment until after their second missed period. If you find this worrisome, speak up! Obviously, if you have any complications, the practitioner will see you sooner, but many women simply want the assurance that everything is going well and that they are taking proper care of their body.

There is something difficult to accept about being pregnant in the early stages. For most women, the earliest symptoms are a missed period and being a bit sleepy. That simply doesn't feel drastic enough to signify a new life growing inside your body. In the beginning of all of my pregnancies, I really felt like I was going to start my period any minute.

ELSEWHERE ON THE WEB

▶ Toni Weschler is an expert at fertility charting, both for conception and birth control. Her book *Taking Charge of Your Fertility* has become the backbone of the fertility world. Weschler also has a Web site (www.tcoyf.com) dedicated to helping you get pregnant, including the use of an online fertility tracking software called Ovusoft. This book and Web site can guide you through everything you need to know to figure out exactly when you ovulate and when you are most likely to conceive.

Early pregnancy doesn't feel like we think it should. After all, pregnancy is about baby movements and huge bellies, right? So if you're feeling a bit surprised at how **not** pregnant you feel, do not be overly concerned. You're in the majority. You can look forward to really feeling pregnant when the other symptoms start, like when you're hanging your head over a toilet bowl.

Waiting for the first appointment can seem to take forever. If you have been eating well, exercising, and taking prenatal vitamins prior to getting pregnant, you're on the perfect course! There isn't really much for you to do in the way of taking care of yourself. I'd encourage you to start reading some great books on pregnancy, birth, breastfeeding, and babies.

Pregnancy lasts an average of 266 days from conception. Most women only have a rough estimate of when they conceived, mainly because sperm can live for days inside your reproductive tract, so we generally call it 280 days from the first day of your last period, or forty weeks (though this assumes that you have a twenty-eight-day menstrual cycle). That makes pregnancy a total of ten lunar months. I think we say nine months to make ourselves feel better.

The About.com pregnancy forum and my e-mail inbox are full of messages asking about the accuracy of due dates in predicting when a baby will be born. About 4 percent of all babies are actually born on their due date. The majority of babies are born one or two weeks on either side of that date.

Due dates are guesses. Even though they don't really predict the day your baby will be born, these numbers are what everyone wants to know. From your parents to your hairdresser to strangers on the street—everyone will ask when you're due.

Medically speaking, counting by weeks is the most accurate way to tell how far along you are in your pregnancy. This is the schedule

▶ *The Official Lamaze Guide: Giving Birth with Confidence,* by Judith Lothian and Charlotte Devries, is an excellent resource for pregnancy and birth. It takes you from before pregnancy all the way until you've given birth. In these pages you'll find everything you need to know to have a safe, healthy, normal pregnancy and birth. This book also supplies practical information on talking to your practitioner and experiencing the confidence you need to give birth to your baby.

your midwife and doctor will go by when taking care of you during pregnancy. A pregnancy is considered full term at thirty-seven weeks, though a normal, healthy pregnancy can go to forty-two weeks.

Because my mother-in-law is such a nervous wreck by the end of my pregnancies, we started telling her we were due a couple of weeks after our real due date. That kept her from freaking out when I went overdue (as I have with all my pregnancies so far). It also kept us sane. We didn't have to field those worried phone calls from her or anyone else because nobody was expecting the baby yet.

Common pregnancy symptoms start quickly. By week 6 of pregnancy, as calculated by the first day of your last period, most women are starting to feel different. I use the vague term "different" because no two women feel the same. You may start to feel the more common pregnancy symptoms, such as nausea, around this time as well. There is no "right" way to feel in early pregnancy—you may have all the symptoms, or only a few.

While having symptoms can help a pregnancy feel more real, don't worry if you're *not* feeling symptoms. You might be one of the lucky women who sails through early pregnancy with nary a feeling of queasiness. This can be perfectly normal.

That said, if you are suffering from pregnancy symptoms that suddenly stop or go away, it is reasonable to request an early appointment with your practitioner. Changes like this can be pinned down to something you're doing to more effectively combat your symptoms, but they can also indicate a potential problem.

Infertility Issues

Infertility is generally considered the inability to get pregnant after one year of having appropriately timed sex without birth control. Infertility is also defined as the inability to stay pregnant, so multiple miscarriages are a form of infertility. About 10 percent of U.S.

ASK YOUR GUIDE

When should I tell people I'm pregnant?

▶ When to tell people that you are expecting is totally a personal decision. Some women decide to tell everyone they can as soon as they know, while others tell no one until they start to show. There is probably a happy middle ground for most women. You may consider your previous pregnancy history and your life situation before you share the good news. Visit my About.com site for more information: http://about.com/pregnancy/bignews.

couples have infertility troubles. While the general definition of infertility is a year of trying to conceive without success, while charting and having sex near ovulation, you may want seek help after just six months. For the majority of older moms, this means about six months of trying to get pregnant. Fertility naturally declines as you get older, so by getting help earlier, you lose less of your potential natural fertility.

Female factor infertility, in which the fertility issue lies with the woman, accounts for about a third of all cases. There are many different types of female fertility problems, including issues related to ovulation, the uterine lining, or structural issues. Testing with the help of a reproductive endocrinologist can help determine the cause of fertility problems. Once the problem has been identified, treatment will likely follow in an attempt to correct the problems found.

Male factor infertility can also be a problem. Male infertility can be caused by many things, including quality or quantity of sperm or a structural issue that prevents the sperm from leaving the body correctly.

Unexplained infertility can be difficult to treat. Some doctors schedule treatment anyway just to see if it works. The treatments you choose will depend on your beliefs about infertility and pregnancy.

Ovulation induction, the usual first step in fertility treatment, uses medications like Clomid to help you ovulate. This type of therapy is to help women who never or rarely ovulate, or who are simply having trouble getting pregnant. Ovulation induction can be done with or without additional treatments.

ELSEWHERE ON THE WEB

▶ Infertility is a huge topic with many different treatments and solutions. The Infertility Guide at About .com (http://infertility.about .com) offers up information on different types of infertility, the latest in treatment for infertility, and stories on the emotional aspects of infertility, like how to deal with a baby shower or the holidays.

Sometimes you are simply told to monitor for ovulation and have well-timed intercourse. Other practitioners prefer to use additional methods of treatment, like the intrauterine insemination (IUI).

Intrauterine insemination (IUI) is a minor fertility treatment. It can be done with or without other medications to influence ovulation. This is done to ensure that the sperm and the egg meet. You will be required to test for ovulation. When you notice that you are ovulating, you make an appointment with your doctor. Your husband provides a sperm sample, which is washed and prepared and is then placed inside your uterus with a small plastic catheter. Then you will wait for your next period. The day your period is due, you may be asked to return to the clinic for a blood pregnancy test or to take a pregnancy test at home.

In vitro fertilization (IVF) is an invasive fertility treatment. Your body is given fertility drugs to help you produce more than one egg during ovulation. These eggs are then collected with a needle, guided by ultrasound.

The eggs are placed in a dish and joined with sperm from your husband's sperm sample. If you also have issues with male factor infertility in which there are poor quality or low quantity of sperm available, an additional procedure known as intracytoplasmic sperm injection (ICSI) can be used to place a single sperm inside a single egg.

In either case, the eggs are then watched for a couple of days and allowed to hopefully fertilize and develop. If the eggs are fertilized and developing normally, they are placed back inside your uterus in a process called a return. You then wait about ten days and take a pregnancy test to see if the fertilized eggs implanted in your uterus. The success rate for IVF is fairly low, though the numbers depend on many factors. Your fertility specialist should be able to tell you your chances of getting pregnant.

TOOLS YOU NEED

▶ As it is a key component to conception, ovulation needs to be monitored. Many fertility doctors want to have at least three cycles charted prior to starting treatment. This can help potentially identify the problem. Ovulation identification can be done using a basal thermometer or ovulation prediction kits (OPK). Once treatment has started, you will likely continue to monitor for ovulation to help aid in your treatment.

Get Linked

For the latest information on trying to conceive and what to do when you find out you're pregnant, check out these additional links on my site to help you navigate the early waters of pregnancy.

OVULATION CALCULATOR

If you need to find out when you are ovulating, or when your due date is, be sure to check out this handy page full of pregnancy and prepregnancy tools.

 http://about.com/pregnancy/pregnancytools

GETTING PREGNANT

If you're looking for the best advice on planning a pregnancy, you'll find specific information on daily life and how to have the healthiest pregnancy possible.

 http://about.com/pregnancy/gettingpregnant

AM I PREGNANT?

Interested in finding out the answers to all of your pregnancy-test–related questions? From how to take a pregnancy test to which pregnancy test is the most accurate, I've got pages and pages of answers to your hottest questions.

 http://about.com/pregnancy/amipregnant

Chapter 2

Prenatal Care:
A Partnership

Choosing Your Practitioner

Choosing your practitioner is a big step. Ideally, you will create a partnership with whomever you choose to guide you through your pregnancy. You should feel completely comfortable sharing personal issues with the person or practice you pick, and on the more practical side, things like office hours should also mesh with your lifestyle and schedule.

It's best to choose a practitioner before you conceive. You may show up for your first appointment already pregnant. If you have already been seeing someone, you may want to reevaluate her services. Many readers tell me that the perfect provider for their annual exam and birth control issues was not a good match to help them through pregnancy.

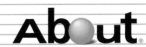

When considering a practice, there are many questions that you need to ask. Here are some examples:

- Is the office conveniently located?
- Do they have office hours that make it easy for me to make appointments?
- Do they accept my insurance?
- Will they make payment arrangements for co-payments or the fees I am due to pay?
- How much time is booked for a regular prenatal visit? Are appointments double-booked?
- What are my responsibilities as a patient in the practice?
- What services do they provide on-site (lactation consultant, lab, ultrasound, etc.)?
- How many practitioners are in the practice? Will I see all of them, or will I have one as my main practitioner? What if I choose not to see one of them because of a conflict?
- How does the call schedule work? How likely am I to get my practitioner?
- How do they want me to contact them in an emergency?

Some women will choose a midwife.   A midwife is someone who is trained in normal birth and who cares for women experiencing a normal, healthy pregnancy. Your midwife may or may not work in conjunction with a doctor.

More and more women are choosing midwives for the personalized care they offer. On average, midwives spend more time with each woman at a prenatal visit than medical doctors do. You are able to build a stronger relationship when your visits do not feel rushed.

Your midwife may be a nurse. Usually these are certified nurse midwives (CNM). After nursing school, a certified nurse midwife

ELSEWHERE ON THE WEB

▶ The My Midwife Web site (www.mymidwife.org) does a great job of explaining what certified nurse midwives and certified midwives are and how they help in pregnancy. The site's "Find a Midwife" search function helps visitors find midwives in their area. The site also offers some great resources, including information you can download about your body after pregnancy, testing for birth defects, and fetal monitoring.

must complete postgraduate work in midwifery at an institution accredited by the American College of Nurse Midwifery (ACNM) and then complete an apprenticeship similar to a medical student's residency. She must also pass a rigorous written and practical exam. ACNM also has a certified midwife program for people without a nursing degree.

Other midwives may have graduated from schools other than nursing schools. Still others study under older, more experienced midwives to learn the art and science of midwifery. Each state looks at midwifery differently. Some states license midwives, while others don't. (See Appendix C for a listing of organizations.)

Obstetricians also take care of normal pregnant women.

An obstetrician is a medical doctor who has chosen obstetrics and gynecology as her specialty. Obstetricians are licensed to practice by individual states but are eligible to apply for that license in all fifty states. The American Board of Obstetrics and Gynecologists (ABOG) accredits residencies, and the obstetricians' governing body is the American College of Obstetrics and Gynecology (ACOG).

You might have the option of choosing to see a family practitioner. Not every family practitioner will see obstetric patients. Some have completed a fellowship in obstetrical surgeries, meaning they are able to do surgeries such as cesarean sections. Others do not perform surgery and must consult with an obstetrician.

Unassisted childbirth is also an option.
Some people believe that no doctor or midwife should care for a normally healthy pregnant woman. These women choose to give birth without any assistance, sometimes not even their spouse or family members.

Who should I see if I have a high-risk pregnancy?

▶ I've counseled many of my clients with high-risk pregnancies to see a maternal fetal medicine (MFM) specialist or perinatologist. After completing a residency in obstetrics and gynecology, this type of doctor completes another program called a fellowship in MFM, making him a high-risk pregnancy specialist.

Where to Give Birth

Where you choose to give birth is a very personal choice. Many women assume that there are no choices in where to give birth. The truth is you always have a choice.

These are the basic issues to cover, no matter whether you choose to give birth in a hospital, a birth center, or at home:

- Location of the facility
- Payment options or plans
- Level of care
- Programs or specialty options
- Providers who practice there
- Insurance acceptance

Other advice for choosing a place of birth includes finding out about each location. Talk to other women who have given birth there or used a particular practitioner. The facility's Web site and promotional brochures will also help you develop specific questions.

Consider taking a tour that is offered by a hospital or birth center, though it is also often recommended that you stop in at a non-scheduled time to see a regular day. This way you can see the facility in action before you make a decision.

Home birth is a popular option for low-risk pregnancies.

There are many reasons why you might decide that home birth is right for you and your family. Sometimes it is the sense of safety and calm you feel being in your own home. Other times it is the ease and convenience of not having to go anywhere in labor.

Home birth is an option for most mothers who are experiencing a normal pregnancy and have no chronic health complications. The final determination will come from a joint decision with your practitioner.

ELSEWHERE ON THE WEB

▶ Vaginal birth after a cesarean (VBAC) can be a hot-button issue when it comes to finding a hospital. You must educate yourself about having a baby after a previous cesarean. The International Cesarean Awareness Network (ICAN) has a great section of handouts on vaginal birth after one or more cesareans. Visit www.ican-online.org.

Midwives are the practitioners that usually attend home births, though some doctors do practice home birth. Who can legally attend a home birth varies from state to state. Be sure to ask an organization that specializes in home birth about the law in your state. Many hospitals and practitioners' offices are not as up to date on the legal status of home birth practitioners.

Here are some questions to ask your midwife or doctor about home birth:

- How long will you stay after the birth?
- What do you bring with you, and what do I need to provide?
- What is your backup hospital?
- What is your home birth transport rate?
- For what reasons do you transport to a hospital?
- Will you stay with me if I need to go to the hospital?
- What emergencies are you equipped to handle at home?
- What do your fees cover (prenatal care, birth, postpartum, etc.)?
- Is there backup if you are not available?
- Who can be with me at my birth? Family? Siblings? Friends?

During labor your baby will be monitored either by fetoscope or Doppler. Your midwife will bring these medical devices with her to your birth. She may also bring oxygen, medications to be used in emergencies, and other equipment for needs like suctioning. Most midwives do not use pain-relieving medication for home births because of the added risk to baby and mom. Instead, they offer a variety of other techniques, including relaxation, massage, hydrotherapy, hypnosis, and whatever else you desire. Your midwife will be able to tell you more and help you find a good childbirth class that will cover the topics you need to manage labor.

ASK YOUR GUIDE

How do I know if home birth is right for me?

▶ My advice is to first look at the home birth options in your area. Interview local midwives or doctors who have home birth practices. They will help you decide if you are a good candidate for home birth, and you can decide whether the option feels safe and right. If it winds up not being the best thing for you, you can at least say you looked at all of your options.

Birth centers offer a bit of both worlds. These are usually free-standing centers where normal, low-risk pregnant women are seen for labor and birth. Doctors or midwives, depending on the center, staff birth centers. The gold standard of a birth center is accreditation by the Commission for the Accreditation of Birth Centers.

Birth centers are known for their home-like atmosphere. Rather than the standard hospital bed, you typically have a queen- or king-size regular bed, complete with comfortable sheets. Most of the birthing rooms have rocking chairs and may also have a water-birth tub or shower. You are encouraged to move around in labor and personalize the space with your own clothes, music, or whatever you would like.

Using a variety of methods available, the nurses or your practitioner will monitor your baby in labor. Medical equipment is available in the unlikely event that you should require assistance.

Questions to ask about birth-center births include these:

- What options do you have available (water birth, showers, etc.)?
- Do you provide a family room for guests?
- What is the average postpartum stay?
- Are you accredited? If so, by whom?
- What do the fees cover (prenatal care, birth, postpartum, etc.)?
- What is the transport rate for your facility?
- For what complications do you transfer care?
- Which hospital do you transfer to? Which practitioner?
- If I go to the hospital, will my practitioner come with me?

Talk to other moms about their births at birth centers. Many are very delighted about the care they received. Birth centers are

ELSEWHERE ON THE WEB

▶ Childbirth Connection developed and carried out a survey to find out what mothers wanted from their birth experience in order to improve maternity care for mothers and babies. Visit www.childbirthconnection.org and search for the Listening to Mothers surveys. You'll also find some of the answers they received and the postings on the site's forums.

very low key and do only births, so there are not many laboring women present at one time, nor are there people who are infectious or very ill. They also usually offer a quieter environment than most hospitals.

Many women still give birth in hospitals. This might be a default option for you, or you may require a higher level of care because you or your baby is ill. If you are ill, or your pregnancy is troubled, a hospital birth is the safest place for you to give birth.

Hospitals realize that for many healthy women, having a baby in the hospital is a choice. Use this knowledge to your advantage when shopping for hospitals and find the ones that are the most flexible and can meet your needs. Remember, you are the consumer. You are paying for the use of their facility and for their services, and you *do* have choices and options.

Here are some questions to ask about hospital birth:

- What do the fees cover (prenatal care, birth, postpartum, etc.)?
- What is your induction rate? Cesarean rate? VBAC rate?
- What is the average stay in the hospital?
- Do you provide tubs for water birth?
- Do you have twenty-four-hour obstetrical anesthesia?
- Do you have a lactation consultant available seven days a week?
- What is your rooming-in policy?
- Who can be with me for a vaginal birth? A cesarean?
- What are your sibling visitation policies?

Be sure to do more than simply talk to people on the phone or read information on the hospital's Web site. Take a tour of the

ELSEWHERE ON THE WEB

▶ The Joint Commission on Accreditation of Healthcare Organizations (JCAHO) lets you search for hospitals by name or zip code and do a quality check of certain procedures specific to labor, such as episiotomy. The JCAHO also rates neonatology care. This might be helpful in selecting a hospital. Visit www.qualitycheck.org.

facility. Many hospitals offer tours after an information night, but you should also consider coming in at a different time to get a more realistic view of what's going on.

Talk to other women who have given birth at the hospital you are considering. Ask what they wanted out of the hospital experience and how closely their expectations matched what they actually got.

What is the right answer for me?   Whether it is a choice between multiple hospitals or the decision to have an out-of-hospital birth or a hospital birth, you may have to do more research.

Look for a place of birth that meets all of your requirements and one that has attractive options. Figure out the most important criteria for you in a place of birth. Once you've ranked these criteria, examine the options individually to see which one measures up.

There are also times when your choices are very limited. In these cases it is best to know what you are dealing with and how to work within the system. For example, if you want to have your baby with you twenty-four hours a day but your hospital does not allow rooming-in, work on this prior to having your baby. Be willing and able to provide them with information on why rooming-in is the best thing for mothers and babies and how medical science backs that up. Remember, these are businesses that exist to help you. They may be out of touch with the most recent research, but any good facility should be completely willing to work with your needs and wants.

Enlist support from other practitioners. You might write to your pediatrician to ask for an exception and to the hospital administrator to ask about the reasoning behind this rule. Any effort to become more educated about your birth options is worthwhile.

▶ Hospitals can now apply for the Baby Friendly designation. The designation ensures that the hospitals are striving to provide the best science and medicine have to offer in taking care of mothers and babies. The standards promote models of care that improve birth outcomes and help produce healthy babies.

Anatomy of a Prenatal Visit

The purpose of prenatal visits is not only to monitor your health and that of your baby but also to allow you to build a relationship with your practitioner and to get your questions answered. Prenatal visits occur at regular intervals during pregnancy.

These regular intervals will change throughout pregnancy, corresponding with certain changes in your body or with your baby's growth. The first question usually pertains to when you will have your first prenatal examination. Many practices will only see you after you have missed two menstrual cycles.

Readers often tell me that pushing this first prenatal exam later in the pregnancy concerns them. When making this appointment, be sure to specify any medications you're taking and to request that someone call you back about their safety during pregnancy.

Your first prenatal visit will usually be the most comprehensive. You will be given a complete physical exam, including a pap smear, breast exam, and blood work. Someone will also take a lengthy personal medical history from you. This person might be your midwife or doctor, or it could be a nurse in the practice.

During the first twenty-eight weeks of your pregnancy, you will most likely be seen once a month. Some visits may be pushed up or back to hit a certain week of gestation, say for a particular prenatal test. But in general, the four-week schedule works well for normal, uncomplicated pregnancies.

At twenty-eight weeks of pregnancy, just as you are entering your third trimester, you will begin to see your practitioner every other week. Again, there is a bit of leeway depending on your health and how the pregnancy is going. Some practitioners also don't begin this every-other-week regimen until slightly later in the pregnancy—say, thirty or thirty-two weeks.

Around thirty-six weeks, your prenatal visits will begin to occur weekly. This will most likely continue until the end of your pregnancy.

ELSEWHERE ON THE WEB

▶ If you're interested in your state's laws regarding birth options and policies, visit www.birthpolicy.org. Whether it's newborn screenings, cesarean sections, or other maternity issues, this site has a wealth of information.

Some practitioners choose to see patients every few days during weeks 41 and 42, so keep that in mind if you go past forty weeks.

After the first visit, you will settle into a routine. A regular prenatal visit will consist of the following:

- Weight check
- Blood pressure check
- Urine screen
- Fetal heart tones
- Fundal height
- Discussion time with your practitioner
- Other tests as needed

If your pregnancy gets bumpy or you have other questions or concerns, you may have a different pattern of visits that might even be spread among different practitioners. For example, you might see the midwife for most of your visits but also see the doctor every so often. You may also occasionally have a prenatal visit with a specialist.

If you have a chronic condition such as an autoimmune disorder or heart problems, you may also need to see your other practitioners. They should be used to working together in the cases of pregnancy, though you should always be sure they are talking to you and to each other. This helps ensure positive communications and good care for you and your baby.

Common Tests in Pregnancy

Once you're pregnant, everything seems to take on a different feel. Maternal instinct kicks in, and you always worry that what's being done is okay for your baby. Don't be concerned that something is wrong every time someone asks for blood or offers you a special

Is it normal to have vaginal exams at every prenatal visit?

▶ Vaginal exams are usually not necessary at every prenatal visit because they do carry risks and are probably not your favorite thing to do. I know that some practitioners will do one or two at the end of your pregnancy just to see what is going on with your cervix. If you are wondering why you're having so many—just ask!

test. Many tests are considered standard during pregnancy, even with a healthy mom and baby.

Blood work is a very common pregnancy test. You will probably have blood drawn at the very beginning of pregnancy. This is your baseline blood work. It will usually consist of a complete host of blood tests, including these:

- Blood type
- Rh factor
- Immunities
- Iron levels
- Thyroid levels
- Infections
- Other tests as needed

Sometimes your first lab work is actually a pregnancy test. This pregnancy test is looking for human chorionic gonadotropin (hCG). Presence of hCG in your blood above 5 mIU indicates you are pregnant. These levels should approximately double every forty-eight hours. For this reason you may have this blood work repeated in a couple of days.

Other blood tests in pregnancy may include the following:

- **Neural tube defects screening:** Between fifteen and seventeen weeks of pregnancy, you may be offered a blood screening for neural tube defects like spina bifida. It may be called an alpha-fetoprotein screening or a quad or triple screen. These are all different types of tests for the same thing.
- **Gestational diabetes:** The most common time to screen for gestational diabetes is around twenty-four to twenty-eight

▶ Having your own pregnancy weeks calculator can help you keep track of pregnancy changes and many other things. While most laypeople like to talk about pregnancy in terms of months, most medical professionals calculate by weeks to be more exact. Consider printing a pregnancy weeks calendar or purchasing a pregnancy wheel over the Internet. Try www.modimes .org or www.amazon.com.

weeks of pregnancy. This is a simple blood test, though they may ask you to alter your diet or completely fast prior to having your blood work done. They will give you a glucose-laden drink and then test your blood to see how well you metabolize the sugar.

- **Glucose tolerance testing:** A step up from the gestational diabetes screening, glucose tolerance testing is done only if your results from the original screening were not within normal limits. Here you will fast, be given a drink of a sugary substance, and then have your blood drawn again three more times. This can also be called a three-hour glucose test.

- **Vaginal swabs (and other swabs):** This is usually done to test for group B strep, also known as GBS or beta strep. Many practices do this late in pregnancy. Group B strep can cause preterm labor, so you may be tested earlier if you have any problems with preterm labor or if you have a history of preterm labor or group B strep. Approximately 30 to 40 percent of women test positive for group B strep, which will not harm them in any manner. The fear is of passing it on to the baby during labor or birth. If you test positive, you will be given intravenous antibiotics during labor.

- **Specialty testing:** This includes fetal fibronectin for preterm labor or certain immunities like rubella.

Urine tests are also done throughout pregnancy. Your urine will be checked at every prenatal visit for various substances. Every practice checks for different things. Some examples are protein, sugar, ketones, leukocytes, and blood. There are also specialty urine tests, like the twenty-four-hour urinalysis, which tests for severe conditions like eclampsia.

Your blood pressure will be routinely screened. Throughout pregnancy, your midwife or doctor will monitor your blood pressure. A slight rise is fairly normal and not considered worrisome. It is when you have a substantial rise in blood pressure that your practitioners will worry. This could be a one-time thing or a trend to watch. Look for this at every prenatal visit.

Ultrasounds may be ordered if you are having complications. Though you might think that ultrasounds are routine for every pregnancy they are not. However, many practices do routinely do ultrasounds. They typically do these as fetal anatomy screenings around twenty weeks of gestation.

I often get e-mails asking how to get around the issue of no routine prenatal ultrasounds. I always try to point out the bright side: If you're not getting ultrasounds, then your pregnancy is on track. Of course, it is also important to talk to your practitioner about why you would like an ultrasound. Most doctors and midwives are happy to help you address your concerns one way or another.

In general, ultrasound is used for complications. For example, ultrasound can show you if you are having a miscarriage, or it can show you where your placenta is located. If you have a history of or reason to be concerned about physical deformity, ultrasound can detect certain problems with some body systems, depending on when it is done during pregnancy. Ultrasound can also track the growth of your baby. It is frequently used in multiple pregnancies to tell the positions of the babies in relationship to the cervix and to look for potential complications like twin-to-twin transfusion syndrome (TTTS).

You might think ultrasounds are a given. An ultrasound may be particularly important to you if you want to find out the gender of your baby. Talk to your practitioner about the pros and cons

ELSEWHERE ON THE WEB

▸ The U.S. Food and Drug Administration (FDA) has sent out warnings about what they call fetal keepsake videos. These are videos of ultrasounds done in non-medical facilities such as shopping malls. These companies, whether run by medical personnel or not, are not your practitioner, and the procedures they perform carry certain risks. See what the FDA has to say about the issue at www.fda.gov/cdrh/consumer/fetalvideos.html.

of ultrasounds in pregnancy. You may also want to see what your insurance company will cover. If you do not have a medical reason, they may not cover the ultrasound. I try to remind moms that if you are not having ultrasounds, it means that everything is going well.

Here are a few of the reasons that ultrasounds are done:

- Questionable dates of conception
- Bleeding
- Previous ectopic pregnancy
- Suspected multiples or history of multiples
- Large or small size for dates
- Question about the baby's position
- Screen for deformities with history or age-related issue

As you can see, the reasons for having an ultrasound are varied. Most are not things you would want to experience in pregnancy. When you interview a practitioner, ask when she does ultrasounds, for what reasons, and what her policy is on ultrasounds without medical necessity. Many practices will allow you to pay for an ultrasound up front without having to worry about dealing with an unlicensed provider (think malls again) and not sweating the insurance payments.

Another thing to consider about ultrasounds is that they do have limitations. For example, while ultrasound may be good at determining the age of your pregnancy prior to twelve weeks, the more pregnant you are, the less likely they are to be accurate for dates. In fact, after twenty weeks you should not even use the "due dates" given by ultrasound because they are no more accurate than your dates by menstrual cycle.

Ultrasounds are not useful for guessing the size of your baby either. Later in pregnancy many people will try to tell you that an ultrasound can tell you the size of your baby, but these are only inaccurate guesses. Ultrasound can be off 10 percent or more in either direction and should not be used for this purpose, particularly when making decisions about labor.

All of the medical reasons aside, you will probably enjoy seeing your baby in an ultrasound. If you are just having a screening without complications, you can usually have someone with you. Some facilities even allow you to videotape the session. You will be given pictures of your baby to take home with you. Be sure to scan them and print them out, as these photos will fade over time.

How to Talk to Your Practitioner

Pregnancy raises many questions. Hopefully you have chosen a practitioner with whom you get along well. Part of the reason for carefully choosing a practitioner is that you will be placing a lot of trust in this person.

Many times moms tell me they are concerned about talking to their doctors or midwives. Do not worry about asking stupid questions or sharing intimate details. Your practitioner is a professional who understands that you are paying money for her time and knowledge.

Also be prepared to do your share. You cannot expect your practitioner to spoon-feed you everything you need to know about pregnancy. You need to explore all of your options and be open-minded as you form opinions. You must educate yourself about what is available and what might work well for you.

Once you have this basic knowledge, you can begin to discuss various issues with your practitioner. What are their common practices regarding a certain topic? When do they use this intervention? What do they request that you know or decide beforehand? Your being able to ask intelligent questions is also appreciated.

Talking to your practitioner need not be difficult. It is usually easier for you to have any type of discussion with your clothes on. Do not hesitate to ask for the opportunity to get dressed before having any conversation. You also have the right to have a conversation while not on the exam table. You can sit in a chair or move into an office rather than sitting on the exam table.

If you choose a practice with multiple practitioners, find out how to deal with information management. I know how hard it can be to explain your wishes to one practitioner, let alone several. For example, one doctor might tell you that it is okay for you to walk during labor. Will all of the partners agree to this as well? During labor is not the time to find out. Is there a way to convey your preferences to all the partners? Be sure to ask the best way to make your desires known to this large group of people.

Be sure to carefully word your questions. Open-ended questions are more likely to give you the answers you are looking for from your practitioner. Avoid asking questions that can be answered simply, or with a yes or no. For example, there is a huge difference between asking "What is your episiotomy rate?" and "For what reasons would you do an episiotomy?" Though they both seem similar, the former gives you a number but doesn't give you the reason. The latter explains why it's done and allows for further questioning. Here are some examples of conversations:

Conversation One
Woman: **How often do you do episiotomies?**
Practitioner: **Only when necessary.**

This conversation doesn't tell you how often episiotomies are performed or for what reasons.

Conversation Two

Woman: What percentage of first-time moms in your practice need episiotomies?

Practitioner: Very few first-time moms need episiotomies—maybe 5 to 10 percent in my practice.

This conversation gives more information and allows your practitioner to provide you with education, should they choose to expound. It opens the conversation up for discussion rather than closing with a simple answer.

When to ask questions may be a concern. Obviously some questions need to be asked immediately, no matter what the time of day or night. These might include the following:

- Worrisome symptoms like bleeding or pain
- Decrease in the baby's movement
- Instructions once in labor

There are also questions that will occur to you as soon as you have walked out of the door from your prenatal appointment. You will also find that as questions bring answers, the answers usually bring more questions. This is a normal part of learning and growing.

To help you remember the questions that come up in between appointments, I recommend writing them down in a notebook. Bringing the notebook with you to your prenatal appointments ensures that you do not forget to get your questions answered. The notebook also gives you a place to write down the answers. If you really want to remember the conversation consider bringing someone with you, like your spouse or a friend.

ELSEWHERE ON THE WEB

▶ "10 Questions Every Pregnant Woman Should Ask" is a very handy document to bring with you to your prenatal appointments. It provides you with sample questions as well as an idea of how to formulate your own. Visit www.mother friendly.org.

Some conversations will worry you. There will be topics that are hard to broach or that you are particularly worried about. This might make these conversations harder. You might be concerned because you are fearful of hurting your practitioner's feelings. You might be concerned about a potential conflict. Or perhaps being pregnant has made you stand up for your opinions and ideas for the first time.

The rules of conversations such as these are simple:

- Be prepared by knowing your topic or how you feel.
- Be calm.
- Be respectful.
- Be sure to listen to the other person or people involved.
- Repeat back to them what they have said to you to be sure you have understood their position.
- State your thoughts, desires, or opinions as clearly as possible.
- Be willing to take time and come back to discuss everything again.
- Avoid making demands.
- Thank the other party(ies) for listening to you and having the conversation.

Mutual respect can go a long way toward resolving any issues or concerns you may have. Having an open mind and truly listening to the other party can also help.

Parting ways with practitioners is tough. This is not an easy decision to come to for anyone. Sometimes it's a timing issue, and the practice is not a good match to your lifestyle. Sometimes the issue is one of money and insurance. There are even times when it is a conflict of opinions or beliefs that previous attempts at resolution have failed to resolve.

It is never too late to leave a practice, though the sooner you do it, the easier it often is on all parties involved, including your practitioner. One of my doula clients made the tough decision to leave her doctor around her thirty-ninth week of pregnancy. She made it to a couple of visits with her new doctor before she had her baby. It was one of the most beautiful births I have ever attended. This mom was thrilled that all of her wishes were respected, though labor was different than she had hoped. She was very glad that she made the difficult decision to leave her original doctor, even so late in the game.

If you decide to leave your current practice, you need to sign a form releasing your medical records to your new practice. You are allowed one free copy of your records for your own purpose, and after that the practice is allowed to charge a nominal copying fee.

I also encourage you to tell your former practitioner why you are leaving the practice. This can be done by phone or by letter. Letting your provider know why you are leaving clears up any misconceptions and allows him the opportunity to make future encounters with other patients different, whether that means accepting different insurance plans, changing office hours, or being more open-minded to options in pregnancy and birth.

You should be able to talk to your practitioner You are placing your life and the life of your baby in her hands. In your partnership with her, you will learn to trust her and value her opinion—and vice versa.

Get Linked

At my Pregnancy and Birth site on About.com, *you can find more information on the issues I've discussed in this chapter. The following links are to articles and resources that might help you.*

IMPROVING YOUR DOCTOR-PATIENT RELATIONSHIP

Here are some tips on nonverbal and verbal communication to evaluate your relationship with your doctor or midwife.

 http://about.com/pregnancy/docpatient

HOSPITAL INTERVIEWS

Here are even more questions to ask your hospital or birth center when looking for the perfect choice.

 http://about.com/pregnancy/hospitalinterview

PRENATAL CARE

Here you'll find more ideas and suggestions to help you during pregnancy.

http://about.com/pregnancy/prenatalcare

Chapter 3

Your Changing Body

Common Pregnancy Complaints

You will find that your body changes rapidly in pregnancy. It may not be the growth of your belly that you expected at first, but there are plenty of changes going on. I found it surprising how sudden—and sometimes how severe—some of these changes were. The good news is that not everyone has every symptom. Even if you've been pregnant before, this time will probably be different.

Morning sickness is not fun. About half of all pregnant women experience some form of nausea or vomiting, frequently called morning sickness (though it can happen at any time of the day or night).

You may not begin to experience any morning sickness until you are about six weeks pregnant. While some moms feel something a little before or after, six weeks seems to be when it starts for most women. So do not hit the panic button if the pregnancy test is positive and your stomach is not churning.

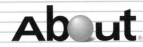

The way you deal with morning sickness depends on what you feel. Morning sickness can feel different from pregnancy to pregnancy and might include slight queasiness, full-blown nausea, or vomiting. I was always more likely to feel nauseated when I was hungry, especially in the morning after not eating all night, and if I got nauseated I was more likely to throw up. For me a good rule was to not let myself get too hungry. I did this by snacking on crackers when I woke up in the middle of the night.

There are many things you can do to try to help you ease the symptoms of morning sickness. Try these on for size:

▶ Seabands are small, flexible bracelets designed to hit acupressure points on your wrist, which theoretically relieves symptoms of morning sickness. They are inexpensive and drug-free, and it certainly can't hurt to try them. Some moms report that they really help, while for others they don't. One mom told me that they worked as long as she had them on, but she'd better be standing in the bathroom when she took them off!

- Stay well hydrated.
- Eat a bit of protein throughout the day and before bed.
- Suck on something. Sour things can be helpful, but so can ice chips or hard candies like peppermints.
- Eat a few crackers before getting out of bed.
- Put ice in your drinks.
- Try relaxation techniques, like taking a few deep breaths.
- Avoid foods that upset your stomach—eat whatever will stay down.

Morning sickness is usually annoying and uncomfortable, but it rarely wreaks enough havoc to damage you or your baby. Still, it's important to find a remedy that works for you. If you've tried everything, your doctor or midwife might prescribe medications to help ease your symptoms.

There is also a severe form of morning sickness called hyperemesis gravidarum. Women with this condition typically throw up multiple times during the day, and are rarely able to keep anything down. If you have hyperemesis, you may wind up losing weight, but more importantly you may become dehydrated. This requires medical intervention, including potential hospitalization.

The good news about morning sickness for most women is that you will usually see an end to it around the end of your first trimester or after about twelve weeks gestation. Sometimes your nausea will hang on a bit longer, but with the exception of hyperemesis, you should start feeling better at this point in your pregnancy.

Frequent urination is usually unexpected. It might be the hormones or the growing uterus that causes it, but the result is the same. Even if you once had the bladder of steel, pregnancy will make you have to go much more frequently.

The really annoying part of urinary frequency is not during the day. At night in the first trimester, when you are so tired, your bladder will still wake you up. This means you can start losing sleep pretty early on.

There is not really a cure for this symptom. You can try to limit fluids just before bed. Some women report that cuts down on nighttime trips to the bathroom. In general, just keep in mind that you'll need to know where the closest restroom is located at all times.

There are many types of breast changes in pregnancy. These changes usually start to happen fairly early in pregnancy though they can vary widely from woman to woman. Some of the changes you might experience include these:

- Breast tissue growth and cup-size change
- Sensitivity or pain in the breast
- Enlarged or darkened areola
- Development of Montgomery tubercles

Some breast changes are more noticeable than others. Some of my clients say that wearing a bra is excruciatingly painful, while

ELSEWHERE ON THE WEB

▶ The Hyperemesis Education Research, or HER, Foundation has a Web site dedicated to helping women with hyperemesis and their loved ones. You will find stories from other mothers as well as tips on dealing with hyperemesis, from common medications and treatments to a section dedicated to those who will help you care for yourself and your family. Visit www.hyperemesis.org.

others say that something firm and supportive, like a jog bra, really helps. For the most comfort, make sure your bra fits well.

The changes in the breasts are caused from your body getting ready to feed your baby breast milk. If you're not feeling particularly sensitive it doesn't have any real bearing on breastfeeding.

The milk you have in your breasts toward the end of pregnancy and the first few days after birth is colostrum. This premilk substance is the perfect food for your new baby and will not run out before the baby is born. It will not hurt you or your husband. You may notice it in the shower, in the cup of your bra, or when you have any nipple stimulation, as during sex or foreplay. You can wear a nursing pad to protect your bra from the leakage. It is also not a problem if you do not see colostrum, as many women do not see colostrum prior to the birth of their baby.

Fatigue comes and goes in pregnancy.   Typically fatigue is an issue in the first and third trimesters. We are talking bone-weary fatigue. With my first baby, the first clue that I was pregnant was not a missed period. It was the fact that after a full night's sleep, I could barely drag myself out of bed to work for three hours. I came home and took a nap from noon until seven that night. I got up, ate, and went back to bed. The pregnancy test I took the next morning was positive!

It is difficult to be motivated to do anything when you are this tired, but there are things you can do to help ease the fatigue. Avoid caffeine, and get some exercise. If you can, take a nap.

Napping can be a double-edged sword. It's hard to nap if you work during the day or have other children at home (though sleeping when the baby sleeps works here). It's also easy to sleep too much, which might keep you from sleeping well at night.

Insomnia is cruel. It may be cruel, but lots of pregnant moms deal with it. It is very hard to be that tired and unable to sleep.

Many of the same treatments for fatigue will help with insomnia. You can also try things like reading before bed or practicing yoga or relaxation techniques. I personally recommend a good book and a warm bath to help ease you out of the day and into sleep.

Bowel issues are part of pregnancy. The hormones that help your pregnancy thrive also tend to slow down your bowels. This means that you are likely to suffer from constipation at some point during your pregnancy. If left untreated, the constipation can lead to pain, nutritional inadequacy, and hemorrhoids.

You can avoid constipation in several ways. The obvious one is through your diet. A high-fiber diet will help maintain good bowel health. This fiber can come in the form of fruits and vegetables or whole grains. Most of the moms I talk to say that breakfast cereal is the easiest way to get fiber in their diet. Be sure that the cereal you choose has at least three grams of fiber for the best results.

Water is also important to your bowels. Staying well hydrated will help you have more regular and softer bowel movements. If you are already drinking six to eight glasses of water a day, try to take it up slightly.

Exercise is also known for getting your bowels moving. It does not have to be daily aerobics, either. Simple walks or short aerobic programs can help in maintaining a good pattern of bowel movements.

To avoid hemorrhoids, avoid pushing your bowels forcefully or straining in the bathroom. If you are having a hard time maintaining bowel health, be sure to talk to your doctor or midwife. Certain medications and even some prenatal vitamins (particularly those with lots of iron) can lead to constipation.

Heartburn can occur at any point, though it is more typical in the first and third trimesters. In the early part of pregnancy, it is usually caused (and exacerbated) by morning sickness. In late pregnancy, as your uterus and baby grow, your stomach is constricted into a smaller space. This forces the stomach acids into the esophagus.

Sitting up after you eat can help a bit. This gives you a bit of time to digest your food, making more room in your stomach. It also can help prevent the acid from going up your throat. I'd also recommend that you don't try to eat just before bed for the same reasons.

Avoiding spicy and greasy foods is also the best practice if you are suffering from heartburn. This should also go for any food that you find increases your discomfort level, which might be totally different than what you would expect, like ice cream.

For days when the heartburn is really bad, there are over-the-counter products you can use. Ask your practitioner if she has a preference. I used natural papaya, in both dried and tablet form, and found it helpful. If you are using a calcium-related product, be sure it contains no lead or talc.

A backache hurts! But there are some very simple solutions to backache issues in pregnancy. The first is posture.

Be sure to stand up straight. After the fourth month of pregnancy, your uterus comes up out of your pelvis and changes your center of gravity. As a result, you might start leaning forward into your belly's weight. This pulls on your back and causes strain and discomfort.

As your uterus grows, your body has to accommodate the strain. Your abdominal muscles and back muscles both work to support your core and weight. When either is strained, the other must work overtime.

Vaginal discharge is common.   Other than seeing fertile mucous as an increase in discharge when you are trying to get pregnant, you probably don't want to know anything about a vaginal discharge. Pregnancy brings a whole new meaning to that term! It is pretty normal to have a mucous-like discharge throughout your pregnancy, though it is usually heavier the further along you are in your pregnancy. The key is that it should never be green or yellow and it should never have a foul smell. If it does, be sure to tell your doctor or midwife right away.

Leg cramps can send you through the roof!   They are very painful. Usually these do not occur until the end of your pregnancy. They tend to happen when you are sleeping or pointing your toes.

Some suggest that a lack of potassium is to blame for the rise in leg cramps. Many moms tell me that eating bananas helped them. This might be an old wives' tale, but if it helps, great; if not, no harm done. Stretching my calves before bed worked best for me.

To stretch your calves, simply face the wall. Step back with your right leg and press into the calf, stretching it and using the wall to support your body. Hold the stretch for a few seconds. Bring your right foot back to the original place. Now repeat the same stretch on the other leg. This should help reduce the number of cramps.

Exercise in Pregnancy

Exercise used to get a bad rap in pregnancy. It hasn't been that long since they really meant confinement when speaking of a pregnant woman. Now many more women are up and moving well into their pregnancies, and the health benefits for both mother and baby are clear.

ASK YOUR GUIDE

What can I do to ease the aches and pains of pregnancy?

▶ Simple things like good posture and proper body mechanics can really help ease the aches and pains. You can also use warm baths and warm packs, like a rice sock. You can also try stretching, or my personal favorite, pregnancy massage!

Exercise helps you feel better. As with anything that improves your health, exercise is no exception. Most moms who exercise in pregnancy report that they feel better and have fewer pregnancy complaints. This is because exercise helps stimulate your body's natural immunities and strengthen muscles that will help support your pregnant uterus physically.

Studies show exercise in pregnancy can have benefits in labor, too. Labor can be shorter and easier if you exercise in pregnancy. You also have a reduced risk of cesarean section. And your body tends to heal faster when you go into childbirth with a healthy body, no matter how you give birth.

I really enjoyed reminding myself about the benefits to my baby. That is what really kept my body moving when I would think, "Why am I doing this?" Babies are shown to be healthier and leaner when their moms exercise. Studies also include a calmer baby on the list of benefits.

Most pregnant women can exercise. Now, we are all supposed to be exercising most days of the week, even in pregnancy. However, you should not exercise if you experience any of the following:

- Preterm labor
- An incompetent cervix
- Active bleeding
- Certain physical conditions, such as placenta previa, or as explained by your practitioner

If you are allowed to exercise, you may wonder what would tell you to stop exercising. The key to when to stop a workout, either for good or for that session, is to listen to your body. You should stop at any sign of pain, shortness of breath, or concern.

Obviously pregnancy is not the time to take up a sport like cross-country skiing, scuba diving, or horseback riding. Sports and activities that pose no risk of falling and don't require a lot of balance are great for pregnancy. I prefer women new to exercise to try something like walking or swimming. Many women enjoy whatever exercise they have been doing before pregnancy, including running.

You can exercise all the way through pregnancy. Many moms tell me that they exercised all the way up to the very end. Some even tell stories of going into labor hours after a workout. Given the benefits of exercise and the increased labor tolerance for those who exercise, you probably wonder why you didn't think of this sooner. Just remember to start slowly, watch your balance—particularly after the fourth month when your center of gravity changes—and to choose comfortable workout wear.

How Your Belly Grows

When you think of pregnancy changes, you probably envision that beautiful round belly that holds a precious new baby inside. And as the pregnancy test turns positive, you want to know when that will be you.

The belly of a pregnant woman grows differently than simply gaining weight. You will usually begin to notice a small mound above your pubic bone first. One of my clients said it looked like someone had slipped a baseball under her skin, but you could only see half of it.

Typically your belly will not look obviously pregnant until at least halfway through the second trimester. Somewhere between sixteen and twenty weeks, you just wake up looking pregnant. Many moms write me to say they seem to have popped out overnight. That is perfectly normal and not a problem.

BEFORE YOUR APPOINTMENT

▶ If you have any concerns about how your belly is growing, be sure to write them down in a notebook to take with you when you go to see your practitioner. Consider asking her to explain to you how she measures you and what she is looking for with each measurement. Sometimes understanding the hands-on reasons will help you be less worried.

From this point on your belly will continue to get larger. This usually happens from the bottom up. Your belly will take on a shape of its own.

If this is not your first pregnancy, you may show sooner. This is because your uterus is less elastic. Second-(or more)-time moms often write to say they popped out really quickly the second time. Some of this has to do with how long it's been since your previous pregnancy and your body type.

The shape your belly takes—and how soon you change shape—is largely dependent on your body type and shape, the way your baby is lying inside you, and your height and weight. Your personal history also influences the way your shape changes. Some women look pregnant all over. Other moms-to-be do not look pregnant from behind.

If you are overweight, you are much less likely to show early. This can be emotionally disconcerting. Be assured that you are pregnant and that your baby is still growing well. It is more a matter of being able to have your uterus show through your clothes. If you find yourself in this situation, be sure to announce to anyone who might ask when you are due.

If you are underweight before pregnancy, you may show more quickly. This is because your body doesn't hide the growing uterus. Remember there is also such a thing as showing before your uterus is out of the pelvis. Most moms don't like hearing that pouch hanging over their pubic bone is really their intestines.

Be careful when trying to compare your belly. I get e-mail almost every day from some worried mom who tells me she doesn't look like her neighbor or her sister. Remember, every belly is different!

The old wives' tales say you can tell your baby's sex by whether you carry high or low or whether you show from the back. These are all harmless fun—not accurate.

I highly encourage you to take pictures of your belly every month, even in the beginning when you do not feel like you're showing. Some of my moms choose to wear the same outfit, like a bathing suit or shorts and a jog bra. This enables you to get a good comparison. It's also fun to measure your waist. Many moms who write me don't want to know the actual number on the tape measure so they use toilet paper squares to measure each month. The changes are fun to look back on, no matter what you use.

Stretch Marks

Striae gravidarum is a fancy word for stretch marks. These two words strike fear in the heart of any pregnant woman. What they are is a breakdown of collagen in the skin.

The skin is normally very elastic. During pregnancy or times of other rapid weight gain, like puberty, your skin has trouble keeping up with the pace of the growth of the skin. This causes a breakdown of the tissues in your skin, leaving the lines we think of as stretch marks.

Stretch marks usually occur anywhere fat accumulates, especially in the following places:

- Abdomen
- Breasts
- Upper thighs
- Buttocks
- Inner thighs

While these are all potential places for stretch marks to occur, you may or may not see them in all of these places. The truth is you can have a wide range of normal for the number and length of stretch marks. I'll have a mom write to say she has an inch-long stretch mark on her abdomen, while another sends a photo

ELSEWHERE ON THE WEB

▶ Plus-Size Pregnancy is a Web site run by overweight moms for overweight moms. Recognizing that women of size have health concerns and other issues in pregnancy, from finding a size-friendly practitioner to having the right medical equipment, this site really has its act together. Visit www.plus-size-pregnancy .org.

of stretch marks covering only the lower half of her abdomen. Remember, everyone is unique.

At first, stretch marks appear as small red lines. They may become darker during the pregnancy. Sometimes they appear to be brownish. The color they are depends on the color of your skin.

About half of all women will get stretch marks in pregnancy. There is a tendency to inherit skin that is more susceptible to these marks. Ask your mom or sisters if they had stretch marks and if so, how badly. You can also look back at your own puberty to see if you got any stretch marks during that period of rapid growth. Your breasts may say yes.

There are some factors that play into helping you avoid stretch marks, or at least reducing them. One of the things that can be very helpful is staying well hydrated and eating well. Properly hydrated and nourished skin is more likely to stretch nicely and not break down as readily. So drink up and eat your veggies!

As the skin on your abdomen stretches, it can also be itchy. This may or may not mean that you are likely to get stretch marks. It is important to keep your abdomen comfortable. Any lotion will do that for you.

The bad news for stretch marks is that you cannot prevent them. If you are destined to get them, you will. These bad boys tend to show up toward the middle to the end of pregnancy.

If this is not your first pregnancy, you may be worried about adding more stretch marks to the mix. Many second-time moms write me to say they were pleasantly surprised that they did not get additional stretch marks in subsequent pregnancies. They say they may have a single stretch mark that "extends" a bit more, but nothing more. This isn't a hard and fast rule. If you had stretch marks the first pregnancy and carry your next baby in a radically different way, you may get more stretch marks. Carrying twins or other multiples this time? Chances are you will get a couple more stretch marks. The good news is that after your baby is born, your stretch marks will fade. At first they appear to be a bit less red. Then they go to pink. From there, the stretch marks become almost white or silvery.

Treatments for stretch marks rarely work. Even if you want to believe in the miracle, there really is not much to do about stretch marks. Be very careful of claims that a product can completely remove stretch marks. Treatments that contain vitamin A are not indicated for pregnancy because they can cause birth defects. These are the most common treatments and are the closest anyone has to a miracle cure.

Miracle creams are everywhere, including the Internet. Be very watchful about what you buy to put on your skin. Be sure to talk to your doctor or midwife before trying some of these products. Besides not removing stretch marks, you want to ensure they don't harm your skin.

There are also chemical peels and microdermabrasion. Trained professionals should do these treatments. The chemical peels use harsh chemicals to take a layer of skin off. The microdermabrasion uses basically a form of sand to also remove a layer of skin.

There is a lot of work going into the use of lasers to remove stretch marks, though nothing has really been found to be super-effective. It may be worth a consultation with a plastic surgeon to discuss the current options and what is on the horizon.

Stretch marks are a cosmetic issue.

Quickening: Fetal Movements

The first time you feel your baby move is called quickening. You are probably looking forward to this joyous moment with great anticipation. You may wonder when it will happen or what it will feel like.

TOOLS YOU NEED

▸ While there are lots of lotions on the market, some sold specifically for stretch marks, I love the smooth-textured body butters from The Body Shop (www .thebodyshop.com). My favorites are blueberry and coconut, but they have many different flavors. What I like is that they come in a very nice container that doesn't leak. You can rub these in yourself or have someone else massage you. Besides nourishing the skin, using these can also aid in relaxation practice.

ASK YOUR GUIDE

My baby moves a lot. Is it going to have attention-deficit hyperactivity disorder (ADHD)?

▶ Many moms write me worried about what their baby's movements mean. You cannot tell if a baby will have ADHD from the type or amount of movement while in utero. Nor can you tell if your baby will be a boxer, soccer player, or ballerina. If your baby's movements worry you in any way, call your doctor or midwife for assurances of your baby's health.

Many of the women who e-mail me say that the first movements they felt were very small. Some use the words "butterflies" or "gas." Many, including myself, were not sure that what they were feeling was the baby moving. Do not worry if you feel this way—it does become obvious after awhile.

You are most likely to start to feel your baby move between weeks 18 and 24. There are many factors that play into when you feel your baby move for the first time, including these:

- The baby's position in the uterus
- The location of your placenta
- How many previous pregnancies you have had
- Your weight
- Your position (standing, walking, sitting, lying down)

Your baby will begin to move long before you can feel it. The movements are so small that it would be next to impossible for you to feel them in the early weeks.

As your baby grows, the movements become larger. These are more likely to be felt. But your baby has to be kicking or moving in an area in which you can feel those movements. If your baby is kicking inward toward your back, you are less likely to feel that than if your baby is turned around kicking toward your abdomen.

Your placenta will find a home in your uterus. It can be in the front of the uterus, called anterior. It can be at the top of the uterus, called fundal. It can be toward the back of the uterus, called posterior. These are all perfectly fine and healthy places for the placenta to be located. Your placenta can also be located over the cervix, called a placenta previa. This is one that you will need to talk to your doctor or midwife about.

Where the placenta is located will also affect what you feel from your baby. If your baby is kicking toward the front but hitting the placenta, you are less likely to feel this movement. The placenta has no sensation of feeling. (Your baby will not harm the placenta by kicking it.) But you can see how the location of the placenta may delay how you feel the baby move and when.

If you have been pregnant before, you are much more likely to recognize this feeling sooner than a first-time mom. That said, every pregnancy is different, as is every baby. Do not panic if your baby does not move in the same pattern as your previous baby.

If you are underweight or slender, you may feel your baby move sooner than a woman who has a few extra pounds. This is simply because it can be more difficult to feel the baby's movements, particularly earlier in pregnancy, through the skin.

You began your pregnancy worried about when you would feel your first movements. The next thing to worry about will be when you will feel the *next* movements. Once you start feeling movements, you will likely continue to feel movements with great frequency and intensity as your pregnancy progresses.

Feeling a baby move is so much fun you probably can't wait to share these movements with your family and friends. This usually takes much more time. Remember, you can feel your baby internally. Everyone else has to wait until the baby is big enough and strong enough to be felt through everything on the outside. This usually does not start until around twenty-four or more weeks into pregnancy.

Be sure to journal the feelings you have about your baby's movements. After your baby is born, it will be really hard to remember the subtleties you experience while pregnant. Did your baby seem to react to certain foods? Was there a time of day when your baby moved most often? Talk about trying to get other people to feel your baby and how the baby moved or didn't and how they reacted. Feeling your baby move is one of the most special parts of being pregnant and the one most moms say they miss after pregnancy.

BEFORE YOUR APPOINTMENT

▶ Fetal kick counts **are easy ways for you to monitor your baby's movements and your baby's health. Pick a time of day when your baby is usually active and count how long it takes to get to ten movements. Record this daily after about twenty-six weeks of pregnancy. Bring this chart with you to your appointment. Your midwife or doctor will let you know if you need to alter your counting in any way.**

Get Linked

Pregnancy includes a lot of aches and pains and physical changes. While I've included a lot of comprehensive information in this chapter, you can find even more details at the following locations on my About .com site.

PREGNANCY ACHES AND PAINS

Need help reliving some of the common discomforts in pregnancy? Here is a list, sorted by ailment, for relief in pregnancy from the most common causes of pain.

 http://about.com/pregnancy/discomforts

STRETCH MARKS AND BELLIES!

If you're interested in seeing what some pregnant bellies look like throughout pregnancy, look no further! My site has a ton of belly photos from every stage of pregnancy, as well as a separate section on stretch marks. So you can see the before pictures and after pregnancy stretch mark photos. This is fun, but don't take it too seriously.

 http://about.com/pregnancy/pregnancygallery

THE PREGNANT BODY

Have more questions about your body in pregnancy? I've got answers for you at the site. From photos and calendars to questions about what's normal and what's not, there are answers to help ease your mind.

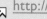 http://about.com/pregnancy/pregnantbody

Chapter 4

Nutrition in Pregnancy

Eating for Two

During pregnancy, you pay close attention to your eating habits. The thought that what you put into your mouth will affect the life and growth of your baby probably weighs heavily on your mind. You want to make the best effort at having a healthy pregnancy. Nutrition is a great place to focus your efforts on staying healthy.

In fact, what you eat has a drastic effect on your pregnancy and dictates how you feel and how well your body finds the harmony of pregnancy. For example, anemia can be tied to your diet.

Women who do not gain enough weight or who have poor diets are more likely to have pregnancy problems. Babies born to these women also have many medical issues. A baby can be born too early and with a greater risk of early death if the mother doesn't eat well in pregnancy. This makes nutrition an important aspect of a pregnant woman's health.

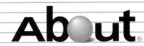

This is one of the reasons that you should never lose weight while you are pregnant. Even if you start out your pregnancy weighing more than you should, it is not wise to lose weight until after your baby is born. The risks you take by losing weight in pregnancy are numerous, including preterm labor, an underdeveloped placenta, and a sick baby.

After your baby is born, there will be plenty of time to lose weight. Breastfeeding, exercising, and continuing your healthy eating habits postpartum can all help make weight loss very easy.

Pregnant women should eat a variety of foods. This should be fairly easy to do these days with the selection of good food readily available and already prepared in many cases. Try to avoid the trap of eating only one or two meals and repeating that meal over and over. While this might be easy on most days, it can lead to nutritional deficiencies, even if the meals you're choosing are nutritionally sound. The reason is because you lack variety.

Grains should make up a good portion of your food, at least seven to nine servings a day. At least half of these servings need to be from whole grains. Don't stress over the thought of nine servings of grains. A serving of grains is just one slice of bread, half a cup of pasta, or a cup of cereal.

You also need three or four servings a day of calcium-rich foods, such as milk, cheese, yogurt, and other dairy, as well as green leafy vegetables, legumes, and some fish. Calcium can prevent iron absorption, so try to avoid iron supplements when having dairy in your meal.

Okay, you probably know that vegetables are also on the list—at least six servings. One serving is a cup of leafy vegetables or a half cup of raw or cooked vegetables. Vegetable juice comes in at three quarters of a cup for a serving, making it not as nutrient-dense as the raw or cooked vegetables. Again, variety is key.

▶ Foods that are as close to their original form are always the most nutritious. For example, a fresh apple has more nutrients than fried apples or even applesauce. Choose fresh fruits and vegetables over frozen and frozen over canned. The same can be said about cooking food. In order, you would prefer raw vegetables to steamed vegetables to cooked vegetables to fried vegetables, as an example.

You need three to four servings of fruit a day as well. Most medium pieces of fruit are one serving. A half cup of chopped fruit is also a serving. Try to eat fresh fruit. Fruit that is coated in syrup adds extra sugar. Dried fruit can be good, but it is easy to eat too much.

Protein, which could be considered the building block of every cell, is very important in pregnancy. In the first trimester, you don't need much extra, but your need for protein does increase in the second and third trimesters. The biggest myth about protein is that it has to come from meat. This is not true.

Protein can come from lean meats, beans, and other sources. You will need about two to three servings in early pregnancy and at least three near the end. A serving is two to three ounces of meat, a half cup of beans or tofu, an egg, a couple of tablespoons of peanut butter or one and one third cups nuts.

Planning your meals helps a lot. By deciding on your meals ahead of time, you can worry less about your eating a nutritious diet. After about a month, it will be nearly automatic for you to plan meals.

You can also learn to shop more wisely by meal planning. This helps get you into the mindset of family meals, too. For fun, try new recipes so you don't get bored, but most of us shop off lists that are pretty stable each week.

You don't need many extra calories. During pregnancy, you only need about 300 extra calories a day. Obviously there are many ways to increase your caloric intake by 300 calories. But the option of peanut butter and an apple is vastly better than a candy bar from the snack machine.

While it is optimal to make every snack a perfectly healthy one, this is not realistic for everyone. Do not stress out over a piece of

TOOLS YOU NEED

▶ Being a vegetarian or vegan in pregnancy is perfectly acceptable. I've found that most people who have become vegetarian or vegan are already pretty responsible for what they put in their bodies. But in case you're looking for help or just good recipes, there are some great cookbooks that also have nutrition advice for you. Try *The Vegetarian Mother's Cookbook: Whole Foods to Nourish Pregnant and Breastfeeding Women—And Their Families,* by Cathe Olsen.

birthday cake or the occasional milk shake. Just try to not make wasted calories a daily habit.

Planning for snacks is probably the best way to avoid eating junk food. In fact, many readers tell me that by carrying their own snacks, they both eat and feel better. Choose snacks that are easy to carry and require little if any work, like fresh or dried fruit, nuts, cheese and crackers, or whole-wheat pretzels.

Keeping snacks handy will help you make good food choices for you and your baby. It is easy to find yourself snacking on fast food or junk from the closest vending machine. Packing a simple snack each day can help prevent you from ingesting extra calories that are more likely to be empty calories, containing no real nutritional value. If your husband wants to help you, try suggesting that he be in charge of helping you pack your snacks for the day.

Let us not forget water! Staying well hydrated will also help with many of the complaints of pregnancy. You will be less prone to constipation and hemorrhoids if your intake of water is good. You are less likely to suffer from headaches if you are well hydrated. Drink between six and eight glasses of water every day.

Water can also help alleviate problems with excessive swelling. The water can flush out your body. This will also help lower your risk of bladder and urinary tract infections, which some women can be prone to in pregnancy.

Cravings in pregnancy are notorious. We've all heard that pregnant women are supposed to crave ice cream in the middle of the night. Or are you sick of the pickles and ice cream jokes yet?

There are some truths to be told about pregnancy cravings. Though some come from a nutritional need, most food cravings are based on hunger. Other women write to say that they knew

▶ Keep a food journal for a couple of days or a week. The point is that if you are honest about everything you eat and write it all down, you can actually get a really good sense of your diet. Take this with you to your next prenatal appointment to allow your midwife or doctor to help you with some nutritional guidance specifically for you. If your practitioner doesn't feel comfortable with discussing nutrition, ask to be referred to a nutritionist.

something was up when they started wanting food that they had previously disliked or hadn't thought of in a long time. Sometimes you can even crave comfort foods for the emotional support you feel when eating them.

Pregnancy cravings are generally not harmful. Heck, if you can convince your husband to go out at 2 A.M. and bring you back anything, go for it! Remember to eat a balanced diet and not have a milk shake every night (just every other night!).

Using Nutrition to Feel Better

What you eat really does affect how you feel. Not only is it the main way for your body to gain nutrients, but it is also a way to help you gain energy and feel strong. The trick is to learn how to eat for your issues.

If your diet consists of mainly junk foods, you will feel it. If you're only eating junk, your body will not have everything it needs to sustain you and your health and to grow a healthy baby. While it is true to a certain extent that your body will shunt many needed vitamins and minerals to the baby, the depletion on you will make all of your pregnancy symptoms worse. You will feel run-down in general, and your outward appearance will also take a hit.

When you are undernourished, even if you are overfed, you will find that you are tired, run-down, depressed, and generally feel horrible. In addition, your hair and nails are weak. Your hair is brittle. You have none of that glow of pregnancy so often talked about.

Anemia is a common pregnancy complaint. By choosing foods that are high in iron, you can help bring your anemia under control without adding an iron supplement and the potential

▶ **We live in an age where bigger must be better. A serving of meat is three ounces, about the size of a deck of cards; a one-ounce serving of cheese is the size of a pair of dice; two tablespoons of peanut butter are the size of ping pong ball; and a serving of pasta is the size of a tennis ball. So when you have a sandwich, two slices of bread is two servings. That glass of milk you drink is more likely two servings. Try weighing your food if you want to watch portion sizes. Remember the kid's meal is usually the appropriate adult portion for meals.**

negative side effects that can go with that supplement. The following foods are high in iron:

- Dark-green leafy vegetables
- Dried fruit
- Whole-grain bread
- Lean red meat
- Iron-fortified cereals
- Tofu
- Blackstrap molasses

You can try to ensure that your diet includes more of these foods. Cereals and whole-grain breads are very easy to add. One mom said she totally turned her iron levels around by switching from iceberg lettuce to baby spinach in her daily lunch salad.

If anemia has been a lifelong struggle for you, simply using nutrition to help raise your iron levels may not be adequate. Even when supplementation is necessary, you must remember that your body will not get everything it needs from a supplement. Instead, proper nutrition is required to help your body most effectively absorb and process any supplements.

What you eat may cause heartburn. It can also be caused by the way you eat. You have probably heard that from your friends; I know I hear it a lot on my pregnancy forums and in my e-mail.

Since the type of foods you choose can be causing heartburn, watch what you eat. Offending foods include anything fried or greasy, spicy foods, and foods with a high fat content. These are often at fault for sour stomachs in pregnancy.

There are other things you can do to help alleviate heartburn. Try staying upright for an hour after eating to keep stomach acids from rising into your esophagus while your stomach is digesting your meal. If you are having problems, talk to your practitioner about remedies like eating papaya, drinking milk, or using over-the-counter products to help alleviate your pain and discomfort.

Weight Gain in Pregnancy

Weight may concern you. A weight gain of twenty-five to thirty-five pounds is considered normal for the average woman pregnant with one baby. You are probably looking at that number and thinking, "Oh my!"

The weight you have gained by the end of your pregnancy is distributed in the following manner:

- Baby: 7.5–8.5 lbs.
- Amniotic fluid: 2 lbs.
- Placenta: 1.5–2 lbs.
- Breast tissue: 1.5–2 lbs.
- Blood: 3 lbs.
- Uterine muscle: 2–2.5 lbs.
- Water: 4 lbs.
- Maternal stores: 8 lbs.

If you started pregnancy below your desired weight, you will want to gain slightly more. A good target to shoot for is about forty pounds.

Various things will affect the weight you gain during pregnancy. Because early pregnancy leaves you feeling green (to say the least), your weight gain might seem to be a bit off as you drop weight early on. Regular illnesses like the flu can also cause your weight to fluctuate. Perhaps you aren't hungry or you're suffering from food aversions. Try not to stress too much about weight gain issues in pregnancy as long as you and baby are doing well according to your practitioner.

ASK YOUR GUIDE

I've heard that a condition called pica can occur in pregnant women. What is this exactly?

▶ Pica is a nutritional deficiency that can happen during pregnancy in which you crave and can actually eat things that aren't food. Sometimes this is a cultural phenomenon, but more often than not it is the body's way of trying to get a missing nutrient. Some women with pica crave fairly harmless substances like ice. Others can crave clay, dirt, burnt matches, or laundry soap. If you ever begin to exhibit the symptoms of pica, speak with your practitioner right away.

How is the weight gain distributed throughout pregnancy?

▶ You will probably not gain very much more than six to eleven pounds in the first trimester. Most of this is water and materials needed to help your baby grow. During the second and most of the third trimester, you will probably gain about a pound a week. Toward the end of your pregnancy your weight gain might slow or cease.

If you are overweight before you got pregnant, chances are you are not looking forward to gaining more weight. You might even believe that you should not gain any weight during pregnancy. Overweight women should still gain a minimum of fifteen pounds. It is a must for a healthy baby.

You have to remember that weight gained in a healthful way is more easily lost than extra pounds packed on by poor eating habits. Pregnancy is not a time to go hog wild and eat whatever you want. Nor should you go on a strict diet or deny yourself treats. It simply means that gaining weight must happen, no matter what your weight was prior to pregnancy.

In certain circumstances you will want to gain more or less weight over the course of your pregnancy. Be sure to discuss with your doctor or midwife the perfect weight gain for you and your body type.

Where will the weight go? Well, the weight you gain will affect the shape of your belly. But the weight won't all go to the belly. Remember that some of it goes to your breasts and your blood stores. Many women report that they feel a bit more in the upper thigh and waist. These stores are for breastfeeding. The calories burned by breastfeeding tap into these stores.

There will be things that affect your weight. Despite guidelines on how the weight gets added in pregnancy, most women tell me that the weight just never goes on the way they think it will.

Things that affect weight gain in pregnancy include:

- Weight prior to pregnancy
- Amount of nausea and vomiting
- Previous medical conditions
- Your eating habits

- Amount of exercise you get
- Your metabolism

Your weight gain will be used to monitor your pregnancy. At every prenatal visit you will be weighed. Your midwife or doctor will talk to you about the weight gain. Anything more than about a pound a week should have you asking yourself what you did differently that week. The answer may be nothing more than a growth spurt or a big celebration in your life. But your practitioner will want to rule out a problem with your pregnancy. Sudden weight gains can indicate a problem that may require further attention, particularly when accompanied by swelling, along with protein in your urine. This is all a part of routine prenatal screening.

Your belly will eventually show. You might show right away, or you might not show until the very end. Is your body type one that makes it look like you swallowed a basketball, or do you get pregnant "all over"? This depends on your body type, heredity, and weight gain. If you have had a baby before, you are probably likely to do the same again this time.

Avoiding Food Hazards

Listeria, salmonella, E. coli—these are some of the food fears that should worry you when eating. The good news is that with common sense you can easily avoid these hazards without sacrificing taste.

Make sure your food is well prepared. This precaution can take away a lot of your risks associated with food during pregnancy. Meats should be cooked well rather than rare or medium rare. If you eat deli or lunch meats out, heat them until they are steaming. This helps to kill potential bacteria inside.

ELSEWHERE ON THE WEB

▶ Food safety is something we're becoming more and more aware of. The problem is that there is a lot of misinformation available on what is and what is not safe in pregnancy. This is too important an issue to leave to hearsay. Food Safety (www .foodsafety.gov) is a government-maintained Web site with the most up-to-date information on what is safe for anyone at any age, including current warnings and general safety tips for foods.

Washing your fruits and vegetables is also important. This will help you avoid illness from pesticides and bugs that can hang out on the skins of these good foods. We keep a small scrub brush next to our kitchen sink just for scrubbing vegetables.

You need to avoid some cheeses. Certain cheeses, mostly those that are mold-ripened or blue-veined, put you at risk. The reason you need to avoid these cheeses is because they have a higher risk of growing bacteria that can cause listeria. However, when any cheese (even those you would normally avoid) has been thoroughly cooked, it is acceptable to eat.

Cheese can be a great source of protein and calcium. So if you like cheese and have it in your diet, you simply need to know which cheeses are appropriate in pregnancy. Since most cheeses are made of pasteurized milk products, most are considered safe for pregnancy and during breastfeeding. Here are some of the most popular cheeses you should avoid in pregnancy:

- Feta
- Brie
- Camembert
- Romano
- Gorgonzola
- Roquefort

There are obviously more cheeses than this that you may need to avoid. Always err on the side of caution when eating cheese that you're unsure of. There will be plenty of time in your life to enjoy cheese, when you're not pregnant.

Not all fish is healthy. There has been a problem in recent years with fish containing high levels of mercury. This can harm your baby during pregnancy. Luckily not all fish is dangerous, but you want to avoid these fish:

- Shark
- Golden/white snapper (tilefish)
- King mackerel
- Swordfish

Fish can be a great source of protein and calcium. The best guidelines are to eat no more than two servings (twelve ounces) of fish a week, only six ounces of which should be canned tuna. Nutritious and safe fish during pregnancy include the following:

- Light tuna
- Catfish
- Pollock
- Shrimp
- Salmon

In addition to foods that you should avoid in pregnancy, there are some common-sense things to know about food preparation. When you are cooking, wash your hands before beginning and after handling any potentially hazardous foods. You should also wash your counters and cutting boards after any contact with raw or undercooked meat. This helps prevent cross-contamination from the raw meat, one of the biggest causes of illness related to food.

Prenatal Vitamins

Hopefully you've been swallowing these horse pills since you made the decision to take the plunge and try to get pregnant. If not, you need to begin taking prenatal vitamins as soon as possible upon finding out that you are pregnant.

ASK YOUR GUIDE

Do I have to take a prescription prenatal vitamin?

▶ The answer is usually no. A prescription vitamin may have something fancy added to it, but a generic pregnancy/lactation-specific vitamin should cover you. If you're in doubt bring in your pill bottle to your next appointment. One potential benefit to the prescription prenatal vitamin is that you are more likely to get prescription coverage for it (though your copay may be more than the cost of the over-the-counter brand).

One of the worst mistakes you can make when thinking about prenatal vitamins is assuming that they will make up for a poor diet. This is not true. You should consider your prenatal vitamin your safety net. It will fill in the small gaps that might occur occasionally.

Take your prenatal vitamins whenever works best for you. Some mothers find that if they take them early in the morning that they feel ill all day. If that seems to be the case for you, try taking your vitamins before you go to bed. This may help reduce your feelings of an upset stomach after taking the vitamin.

There are a couple of things to keep in mind when trying to decide if your prenatal vitamin has everything you need. First, it should have less than 10,000 IU of vitamin A and at least 400 mcg of folic acid. Second, remember that no prenatal vitamin will contain all the calcium you need.

Prenatal vitamins aren't always the easiest pills to take, particularly if you're suffering from nausea and vomiting. Consider switching prenatal vitamins if you're having an issue with your current vitamin. Your practitioner might suggestion a chewable version or a prenatal vitamin with a coating that makes it easier to take. Some practitioners even recommend some version of children's vitamins to help ensure you're getting your essentials.

Some mothers tell me that the taste or texture of their prenatal vitamin makes it difficult for them to take. If you also find this is true, do not hesitate to talk to your midwife or doctor. It is usually no problem to change prenatal vitamins, particularly if it's going to make you feel better.

Since we're on the subject of supplements, did you realize how much of your food is already fortified? Many of the grains you eat these days, from bread to breakfast cereal, are fortified with folic acid. This means that you can enjoy your cereal every morning knowing how good it is for you and baby!

Get Linked

What you eat is what builds your baby. Your diet is a vital part of your pregnancy and your future health. Learning to eat well starts now! For more information from my About.com *site, check out the following links to recipes and more.*

NUTRITION IN PREGNANCY

If you're interested in staying up to date about the latest in nutritional information and nutritional safety in pregnancy and breastfeeding, I've got that information here in a various collection of articles.

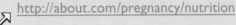
http://about.com/pregnancy/nutrition

WEIGHT GAIN IN PREGNANCY

A huge concern in pregnancy (no pun intended) is the amount of weight you gain and how to avoid gaining too much while still getting enough of the right foods.

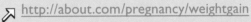
http://about.com/pregnancy/weightgain

SOME PREGNANT WOMEN CRAVE PICKLES.

Here's a guide to some food cravings in pregnancy, from helpful to harmful to just plain annoying. So do you crave pickles? Or is it something else?

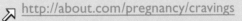
http://about.com/pregnancy/cravings

Chapter 5

The Emotional Side of Pregnancy

Trimesters of Emotional Change

How you feel emotionally in pregnancy is just as important as how you feel physically. The emotional changes are a part of becoming a parent, whether for the first time or the tenth. This doesn't make it fun or predictable.

We often hear talk of the hormones in pregnancy causing mood swings. This can be true in every trimester. Progesterone and estrogen are these hormones.

The first trimester is about acceptance. Other than a couple of symptoms and a line on a small piece of plastic known as a pregnancy test, you have to take your pregnancy on faith. That can be very difficult to do emotionally.

One thing that surprises many mothers-to-be is that even when a pregnancy is planned, even when it took fertility treatments

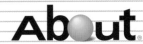

to get there, there is a state of shock. You may find yourself questioning your decision to have a baby and wondering if it was a wise one. Perhaps you're worried about providing for the baby or your life.

No matter what you are concerned about, these feelings are normal. Sometimes you may even feel periods of depression in early pregnancy. You should mention these feelings to your midwife or doctor, who is concerned with your emotional as well as your physical health.

Other emotional changes are common in early pregnancy, including these:

- Excitement over expecting a new baby
- Nervousness about being pregnant
- Confusion at changing emotions
- Disbelief that you are actually going to have a baby

The second trimester is about confidence. Because you tend to feel great in the second trimester, physically you are not as drawn as the first trimester. Your pregnant belly is starting to grow. Even if it is not obvious to everyone outside your immediate circle that you are expecting, the physical changes seem to cement the emotional attachment to pregnancy.

Feeling the baby move makes the pregnancy more real for many women. A couple of moms have written me to share that they really had just been "pretending" to be pregnant until that point. The movements just made it so real.

During this trimester, you might feel any of these things:

- Relieved to feel physically better
- Excited about the baby's movements
- Concerned over relationships with your partner and others

The third trimester is about change. At this point in pregnancy you are starting to feel the pressure of the end. What once seemed nine long months in the distance is suddenly just a few weeks away from being realized. You may find yourself consumed with plans for your baby and new life.

From taking classes to more frequent visits to your midwife or doctor, everything is about your baby now. Your concerns may shift from pregnancy to labor and birth, breastfeeding and parenting. Here are some common emotional themes of the third trimester:

- Obsession with all things birth and baby related
- Fears about labor
- Excitement about meeting your baby
- Curiosity about how your life will change

Building Confidence in Your Body

Confidence in your body is one of the most important things you can have in pregnancy and birth. Unfortunately we have built a society that is terrified of pregnancy and birth. This only makes it harder to have the faith and confidence you need in your body. There are a couple of simple things you need to do to have an emotionally healthy pregnancy.

Trust your body. This sounds simple, right? It should be. Your body was designed to give birth. You were born with everything you need to give birth. Your baby's body is designed to be born with ease.

We like to talk about women who give birth in the fields and go right back to work after slinging the baby on their backs. The good news is that while we don't have to give birth in the fields, we do have the same bodies. The hormonal and physical dance

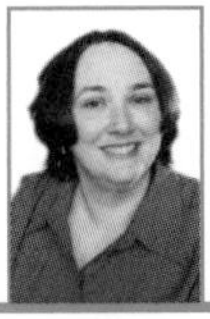

ASK YOUR GUIDE

Since becoming pregnant, I feel like the slightest thing could cause me to burst into tears. Is this normal?

▶ Bouts of crying are common in pregnancy. Sometimes these tears flow for unknown reasons, even to the mother-to-be. I'll admit to crying at a car commercial because it was just so great that we exported cars. Totally irrational. Now we have all those really sweet commercials and we're doomed as pregnant women. Don't panic about crying fits as long as they are not the only emotional state you experience.

▶ **Birth affirmation cards are a great way to help you build confidence. These are positive affirmations that you place around your life where you can see them and repeat them. You can buy these, but it also works to write your own affirmations on blank index cards. Consider affirmations like these: Pregnancy is normal. My body knows how to give birth. I will be a good mother to my baby.**

of labor is an amazing thing to watch. When left alone, the body proceeds unimpeded to open and give birth to a baby.

Any interference with the labor or birth sets off a chain of reactions that can alter the process. This can be a physical intervention or a mental or emotional interference. Interventions in labor as simple as confining a laboring woman to bed can lengthen her labor and cause more pain. Some medications are designed to cause a change in the pattern, such as those medications that are meant to speed or slow labor. Even with the desired change, they may alter labor in ways that are not expected or helpful.

Mental and emotional changes can affect labor as well. This includes fear or worry. It can be fear of the process, of hospitals, or becoming a parent. It can be concern over your health or the baby's health, or about those supporting you. Prevention is the key here, and having that faith in your body goes a long way to helping you.

The fear-tension-pain cycle is often talked about in regard to labor and birth. When you are fearful, you tense your body. When you tense up, you have pain or increased pain. When you have that pain, your body says, "Ah ha! I was right in being fearful!" And the whole process keeps repeating itself in a self-fulfilling prophecy. The key is to try to break into this circle by getting at all of the problems.

Address the fear with knowledge and familiarity. Take a tour of where you will be giving birth and talk to those who will support you. Learn about the process of birth. These are all things known to decrease fear in most people.

Respond to pain in labor. Move your body to assume positions that are more comfortable. Use massage and counterpressure to help alleviate pain.

The release of tension has a lot to do with addressing fear and pain. Relaxation can go a long way to helping to relieve tension in your body. Remember to try to spend time with people who support the positive views of pregnancy and birth that you do. Don't get caught up in reading a bunch of negative birth stories or hanging out with anyone who wants to spend time bringing your sense of normal pregnancy down. Try to find an easy way to get out of these negative situations whenever possible.

Let your body be your guide. Most of us are aware of the cues our body sends. We may refer to them as instinct or an inner voice. Learning to listen to and trust this instinct is key to a normal pregnancy and birth. The beauty of this is that it lends itself to learning to follow that intuition in parenting.

The next time you hear that voice, do not ignore it. Listen to what it says and try to think about what it means. Is it telling you something you already know but choose not to follow? For example, do you know you need to eat more protein? Are you ignoring a nagging concern that you should call your midwife or doctor about?

There are so many times when that nagging feeling has led pregnant women to seek care. One such mom told me that she had read on my site about preterm labor. She really felt like that what she was experiencing. Her doctor told her over the phone she wasn't in preterm labor. This mom refused to listen and went to the nearest emergency room, only to find out that she was in preterm labor, which was successfully stopped because she sought care early. She said despite her doctor's assurances, she knew that something wasn't right. She was able to carry her baby to term because she followed her body's lead and listened to her intuition.

Appropriate and adequate support is crucial to having the faith in your body. You must surround yourself with those who feel as you do. This doesn't mean you exclude yourself from other discussions, but if people want to say negative things that are not framed in helpful ways, you do not have to listen.

▶ If you're having one of those days when you feel uncomfortable in your own skin, try doing something fun and lively. One suggestion that works well is to try finding something that makes you feel sexy and turn it on for your honey. You're both likely to wind up having a great time and you'll turn your thoughts around to something more positive—like the attractiveness of your body and the love for your mate.

There is a huge difference between telling you something as a lesson to help you and telling you something just to rant. An example might be my telling you that I found myself very aware of the peaks of my contractions. This was helpful to me because I knew I was on the downhill slide. But I could tell that story in a different, negative way and have it be about the pain, not the lesson or the benefit.

Announcing Your Pregnancy

Spreading the good news about a new baby is always fun! Seeing the faces of your loved ones as they realize their lives are about to be enriched by another new being is amazing and hilarious, depending on how you share the news.

Are you someone who can't keep a secret? Then maybe you will be the one who chooses to go out and share your good news with everyone you meet. Other mothers-to-be choose to be a bit more selective about whom they tell. You may choose to tell only close friends and family first, saving your boss, coworkers, and others for later in your pregnancy. My husband and I agreed not to tell anyone for a while during one of our pregnancies. The hilarious thing was he would tell complete strangers about the baby randomly. He just couldn't keep the good news to himself.

If pregnancy fears are bothering you so much that you can't enjoy the pregnancy or you're worried that you'll tell someone you're pregnant and then lose the baby, you may delay announcing your pregnancy. This delay is not cause for concern or alarm. Telling others you are pregnant is a personal decision. And once you've told people, there is no going back.

Sometimes your announcement isn't met with matching enthusiasm. That can be really hard on you, particularly if you were not expecting to hear negative feedback. Even if the other person is reacting out of shock or concern, it is still something that

ELSEWHERE ON THE WEB

▶ Telling your boss you are expecting is probably not something you are looking forward to doing. The good news is that it doesn't have to be something big or formal. Ann Douglas offers some wise words on telling your boss about your new bundle of joy; you can find her article online at www.allaboutmoms.com/allaboutmoms/tellingtheboss.htm.

makes you take a step back. Don't get overly concerned about anybody's reaction. The best way to deal with this is directly. Simply look at the person and tell him or her how you feel: "I'm happy about this, and I hope that you can be happy for me." Leave it at that and end the conversation.

Boy or Girl: Do You Want to Know?

Let's face it: the technology is available to find out before birth whether your baby is a girl or boy. A large percentage of people choose to find out. You do not have to be one of them. Amniocentesis and ultrasound are two of the more common ways you can figure out the gender of your baby. Chorionic villus sampling (CVS)—more invasive genetic testing done via needle withdrawal of cells from the villus through the vagina—is also an option.

Genetic testing is more accurate in making the call as to the gender of your baby because it is based on a chromosomal analysis. However, these tests also pose more risk to your pregnancy and may not be worth the risk for most parents unless they were doing the tests for other reasons.

Ultrasound is less risky and more widely available. The accuracy of the ultrasound depends on several factors including the age and position of the baby, the technician's skill level, the machine used, and other factors. This can lead to more surprises at the time of birth.

What do you do if one of you wants to know and the other doesn't? Perhaps you want to know about the baby you're carrying but your husband doesn't—what's a woman to do? The answer is to talk it out. Explore the concerns you each have about the issue. Why do you want to know? Why does he not want to know? Is there a way to find a common ground?

When we were expecting the twins, I knew that with all of the ultrasounds I would have, I would eventually figure it out, being in

ELSEWHERE ON THE WEB

▶ Looking for another fun quiz to help you predict the sex of your unborn baby? Visit www.childbirth.org/articles/boyorgirl.html. These old wives' tales are hilarious and really make you question what you do in your everyday life, as well as what the heck these old wives were thinking. Just answer a few of these questions, like which piece of bread you prefer, and the site predicts whether you'll have a boy or girl.

▶ Reading birth stories is a great way to gather the confidence you need to give birth. I love reading the birth stories that are interwoven in *The Official Lamaze Guide* by Lothian and DeVries. It's nice to read birth stories that don't scare you out of your wits.

my line of work. So I just figured I'd rather know now. My husband did not ever wish to know until birth. So I found out and simply told no one. This was very hard. I really had to check myself every time I argued for a name or bought an article of clothing. In the end the joke was on me. After multiple ultrasounds through my pregnancy said two boys, I gave birth to healthy, identical twin girls.

There really is not a right answer to finding out or not. Doing what is best for you is most important. You may choose to find out with your first child, but not subsequent children or not your first child, but only subsequent children. Or maybe you won't find out any pregnancy and choose to be surprised.

Do you share the news with everyone?   A growing trend I'm finding is that even if couples know the gender of their baby-to-be, they are not sharing as often. They enjoy keeping the knowledge between themselves and letting the grandparents and friends have fun guessing. One mother wrote me to explain that sharing this information with just each other kept the baby very special between them for their pregnancy. She said she felt like they could grow together with this knowledge before having to give part of the baby up to others.

Common Pregnancy Fears

Pregnancy can be a time of worry. I get many e-mails each day about concerns women and men have about pregnancy, birth, and parenting. You need to look at these worries not as flaws but as areas of growth. They are often questions that have not been answered. Addressing your concerns with facts and dealing with them face on is usually the best way to deal with the issues.

Will my husband hate my body?   This is a concern I hear voiced a lot. As women, we worry about our pregnant form versus the model on the cover of a magazine—there isn't a comparison. Dads tell me that the pregnant form of their wives is very sensual. The majority of dads report that a pregnant belly is something that just attracts them. After all, it's their baby!

What if I lose it in labor?   The term "losing it" is something that comes up a lot in my childbirth classes. It really is not one thing, but rather the definition of a loss of control for any one person. Do you worry about losing control in labor and being naked? Maybe your worry is that you will scream? These are normal concerns. The hard part is that labor is a loss of control in so many ways. Try not to think of it as a loss of control. Try thinking of it as a different part of your mind and body taking that control, the part of your body that inherently knows how to give birth. Educate yourself on the specifics of your concerns, be it how to best cover your body (I recommend a jog bra) or what the deal is with vocalization in labor.

What if you never get your body back?   Rest assured, you will one day again be the only one to inhabit your body. It can be hard to remember that when your body is filled with another human being. The kicks and pokes, the aches and the pains all say that your body doesn't quite belong to you.

The good news is that once the baby is born, your body is yours and yours alone. The bad news is that your body is different. Not bad, just different. The added weight that sustained the pregnancy and kept your baby healthy will come off. With a bit of exercise and watching your nutrition, your body will bear only small signs that it once shared space with your miracle.

What if I'm not a good parent?   Many of us worry about this, whether we say anything or not. Translate what this means to you. What are your specific parenting concerns?

▶ A great book that really helps you tap into that inner strength and wisdom is *Birthing from Within,* by Pam England. This book is all about tapping into the inner wisdom that pregnancy brings to you. I love the art projects throughout that help you think of your body, baby, and pregnancy in a totally different way. The small projects for doing things around your home to prepare and get in touch with your partner are great no matter what kind of birth you have.

Will worrying hurt my baby?

▶ Worrying about worrying is a common fear. The good news is that simply being a bit worried, even if it feels like you worry about everything, is not harmful to your baby. Now, constant worry that leads to things like panic attacks, poor eating, or little sleep is something that can be potentially worrisome to your midwife or doctor. Be sure to talk to your practitioner about getting some support to help ease your fears.

I would encourage you to make a list of the traits that belong to the parent you want to be. Are these things you already have? Are there ways to get these skills or traits? Can you read a book, take a class, or listen to other wise parents? No one has the corner on the market for good parenting.

For some moms, the "good parent" fear translates to a larger fear of failure as a woman and mother. We are surrounded with these ideas of a supermom. The truth is you can't have it all, at least not all at once. Some days you'll have most of it, but there is always something else out there. So pick your battles, choose the things that are most important to you, and go for it.

Will something go wrong?   This is a variation on the loss of control. And there is only so much you can control. You can eat well. Plan for pregnancy. Take your prenatal vitamins. See your doctor or midwife. But sometimes there is nothing you can do to prevent something from going wrong. It's not your fault. There is no one to blame.

Sometimes you need to simply have faith that if something goes wrong, you will be able to deal with it. One mother told me how freeing that felt to think of it that way. When knowledge and prayer hadn't worked to alleviate her fears, she found that seeking the wisdom to "let it go" would work, and it did.

In the end, I'd personally recommend that you avoid things that make you worry unnecessarily. More than one woman has written me to say that she was reading a pregnancy book that scared her. There is not a book that is worth reading if it is scaring you.

The Emotions of Prenatal Testing

Prenatal testing is supposed to provide us with answers. These answers were designed to help us get rid of certain worries, most commonly about the health of the baby. It does not always work that way. Now I find that women worry about prenatal testing a lot. What will the test say? If the answer is bad news, how will I handle it? Will I be able to deal with the news? What if the answer is good news? How can I trust that it is accurate?

It is also not simply a matter of hearing positive results. In this day and age of informed consent, we know that we have the option not to take a prenatal test. So now, not only do we worry about the test results, but we also worry whether we should have the tests in the first place.

One mother wrote me a very poetic note about how she hadn't realized how worried she had been until her results came back that everything was fine with her baby. She felt like she was finally able to let go and accept the pregnancy and the baby. This was totally unexpected for her.

Other parents aren't so sure about testing. With my first pregnancy, the doctor I was seeing made it seem like everyone did the screening for neural tube defects, so I just did it. Everything was normal, so in my next pregnancy I didn't question it. Suddenly my world was upside down as I was being forced to consider more invasive testing after an abnormal result. I had never even taken the thought that one step further because I fully expected everything to go as before.

What if you are over thirty-five?   Should you have genetic testing? Seeing a genetic counselor can help you put your risks into perspective. This person sits down with you and looks at all of your and your family's medical history on both sides. He talks to you about social and environmental risks and eventually breaks it down into what the risks really are for you, as opposed to vague numbers for a general population.

A client of mine was thirty-four when she got pregnant. Her husband talked her into seeing a genetic counselor because he

ELSEWHERE ON THE WEB

▶ Sometimes what is bothering you is a previous birth experience. If you had a very hard pregnancy or a difficult birth, this can influence how you feel about this pregnancy. Sheila Kitzinger, a famous birth anthropologist, talks about how previous births affect your experience and how you can help alleviate fears. Visit www.sheilakitzinger.com/ArticlesBySheila/BadBirthHaunts.htm.

really wanted to do genetic testing, figuring if thirty-five was good, thirty-four was close enough. Going in, they both had this thought that their chances of having a baby with a genetic problem was very high, like one in ten. They both left very reassured by the numbers and had an easier time making their decision.

There are not easy answers to these questions. The decisions you make need to be right for you and your family. Try not to be swayed by what others do or say.

If you are getting pressure from your practitioner, ask her why. Perhaps she is only making the offer out of habit. However, just because it's normal practice for her, it may come across as more forceful than she intends.

Working Together

Pregnancy can be a time when couples grow closer together. It is a time to share the hopes and dreams for your future and your growing family. Communication is the key.

Sex is an area most couples share concern over. Continuing your sexual relationship in pregnancy is fine for most couples. But the emotional hurdles may be larger than your growing abdomen.

There are a very few times when sex is not a good idea, like if your water is broken, you are in preterm labor, you are bleeding, or there are other hazards to the pregnancy itself. These issues are usually very obvious, and your practitioner will warn you against sex.

The issue here is more than physical sex; sex is an attraction and a relationship. As your body changes, you may worry that your partner no longer desires your body—or worse, is turned off by it. Most dads say that this is far from the truth and that they still want you. Their problem is that they have emotional issues going on as well, like how can they provide for you and will they hurt the baby if they touch you.

Talking about your concerns with physical contact in pregnancy can be very beneficial. For example, in the first trimester if your breasts are sore, say so! Don't wait until you're writhing in agony and he's left wondering what he did wrong.

Finally, have a sense of humor. There is nothing like making love to your husband and having someone else kick you both. Your sense of humor will also help you in the early months of parenting.

Your relationship is changing. When you met and fell in love with one another, life was more simple. It was simply a man and a woman in a relationship. As your relationship grew you added other players, like your family and friends, but these were grownups who didn't require much attention.

Adding a baby to your lives adds the additional strain of becoming parents. During that first pregnancy, you really have to spend time working through the emotions of becoming a parent and watching your spouse become a parent too. This is where you get to ask yourselves those hard questions, like "What kind of parents do we want to be?"

Being a parent is a constantly evolving process. It can be very easy to make decisions about how you would handle specific situations before you are actually in them, so don't stress over having exact plans.

Watch other parents with their children. Notice what you like about their style. See things you would do differently? That's okay too. Be sure to continue the discussions as the pregnancy progresses and as your children grow.

BEFORE YOUR APPOINTMENT

▶ Before agreeing to prenatal testing that your practitioner feels is routine, ask yourself some questions. What is this test? What can it tell me? What can it *not* tell me? What will I gain from having the information from this test? What will I do based on the information from this test? Your answers may help you make up your mind about doing the tests or looking into less invasive options.

Get Linked

There are a lot of things to think about in this chapter. The links below will cover these topics in depth and answer more of your questions or just allow you time to share with others.

SEXUALITY IN PREGNANCY

Interested in learning more about the emotional and physical changes of pregnancy and how they influence your sex life? Here is a great list of resources and answers to your most common questions, even the ones you were embarrassed to ask.

 http://about.com/pregnancy/sexuality

SECOND PREGNANCIES

Everything is all about the first-time parent. Not so! Here are some articles on pregnancy after your first baby, including issues with siblings, such as whether they should attend the birth, how to make your older child feel welcomed when a new baby is born, and lots of other resources.

 http://about.com/pregnancy/secondpregnancy

SHARING WITH OTHER PREGNANT MOMS

Interested in hearing what other pregnant moms are talking about? Share your fears and concerns along with pregnancy stories at our forums.

 http://about.com/pregnancy/forum

Chapter 6

Beauty and Fashions

Maternity Clothes

Maternity clothes didn't used to be known for their beauty or style. Thankfully the world of fashion has changed. Things have changed drastically even from when I had my first baby nearly fifteen years ago. That is good news! Now you can feel free to shop for maternity clothes that express your individual taste.

Wondering when to wear maternity clothes?   Don't grab for the maternity clothes too soon. Buying clothes too early means you're probably going to buy something a bit bigger than you'd need it, thinking you'll grow into it. The problem is you could also underestimate and wind up having nothing that fits in the last few months. Not to mention the fact that you'll probably hate the sight of the same clothes after eight months.

Your first few pieces should just be clothes that are larger than normal or expandable in some way. These clothes are also helpful to have around for your immediately postpartum body. This leaves

▶ If you are having a problem with backache or pelvic pressure, consider using something to support your abdomen. This is particularly helpful if you are pregnant with twins or other multiples. There are several kinds of support available, including the Prenatal Cradle and the Belly Band. The bigger the product, the more support you have, so keep that in mind when thinking about which one is best for you. If your practitioner will write you a prescription for one of these support devices, your insurance might pick up part of the tab.

you to buy some true maternity clothes when you have a more realistic sense of what you need.

Between four and five months along is an average for when women start to move into maternity clothes, but you can wear them whenever you need the room to grow. When that time is will be different for different people. For example, I usually wear workout pants and pajama bottoms around the house. I didn't have to do anything different for my entire pregnancy when it came to lounging around at home. My work clothes, however, were a different story. Around fourteen weeks into my pregnancy, my pants started to get tight. I moved from my regular dress pants into skirts and pants with elastic. The shirts were still fine. Eventually the belly took over around twenty weeks, and I went to mostly maternity clothes.

If you have baggy, loose-fitting clothes with lots of elastic, you may never need maternity clothes. If you have tailored clothes, you're likely to need maternity, or at least bigger, clothes sooner rather than later. For comfort, I would recommend that you have at least a few maternity outfits.

Maternity clothes have a couple of different ways to incorporate the belly. Some pants or skirts have a stretchy fabric panel that allows your belly to fit inside the pants. This panel expands to fit the size and shape of your belly comfortably.

You can also choose low-rider bottoms that come around underneath your belly. A few styles offer areas that stretch on the sides, but these are harder to keep up around your waist. One mom said she just wore her regular pants most of her pregnancy by using rubber bands threaded through the button hole and looped over the button. This allowed her room to grow. She would wear a maternity shirt or large shirt over the pants to hide the rubber band.

Color is currently in style. Pick colors that go well with your skin tone and eyes. Consider having your colors done at a local department store. This will help you make color choices that are best for you, whether you are pregnant or not.

Patterns are also popular on clothing, but don't overdo it. Pick patterns that flatter your body type and outfit choice. Worried about wide hips? Wear solid bottoms with a brighter color or pattern for a top. Want to minimize your breasts? Try big earrings and solid color shirts. Also, avoid jewelry hanging down into your cleavage. And a word to the wise: Horizontal stripes are never flattering on a pregnant woman.

Remember that being pregnant doesn't mean that you have to drastically change your style. You can still choose very similar styles to what you are accustomed to wearing. If you haven't been a low-rider, belly-baring type of dresser before, you don't have to start now.

Don't spend a ton of money! You could easily spend thousands of dollars on maternity clothes. Even though there are some adorable outfits out there, try to concentrate on what you really need.

My recommendation is to buy some basics and then add on or accessorize to expand your wardrobe. For example, buy a couple of pants and a skirt or dress. Some suggest that you choose a single neutral color, like black, gray, or brown for these basic pieces. Then buy a couple of solid color tops. Mix and match these pieces to make your wardrobe stretch. For fun, add fancy scarves or jewelry to brighten up any outfits. After the basics you can add a couple of specialty items to your closet.

You can shop anywhere. Maternity clothes are cropping up everywhere. You are no longer relegated to the fancy maternity-only

ELSEWHERE ON THE WEB

▶ Pregnancy Fashions (www.pregnancyfashion.com) is a Web site that offers some great advice on all aspects of pregnancy and maternity fashion. Browse their topics or look through their collection of links for a wide variety of information on finding the perfect clothes for you. I love all the pregnancy T-shirts with attitude!

stores in the mall. Now you can find maternity clothes in many department stores, discount chains, and in consignment stores.

One mother told me that she spent much less money and had much more fashionable clothes by avoiding the maternity stores and departments. Her trick? She shopped in the plus-sized section. While these clothes do not work for everyone as maternity alternatives, it's definitely worth a try.

When considering what to wear, don't forget to look in your other half's closet. Your husband probably has a couple of shirts that would work well either as stand-alone shirts or as something over a T-shirt or tank top. Button-down shirts work really well here. You might even give his pants a try, too.

Shoes matter in pregnancy. In addition to the blossom of your belly, you may find that you're a bit off balance, particularly after the fourth month of pregnancy. My advice is to skip the stilettos. Pumps and low heels are fine for short stints, but your basic flats and a nice pair of tennis shoes are also a must. One thing to keep in mind is that your feet can actually grow in pregnancy, sometimes as much as a size! So if your shoes feel tight and it's not from swelling, try going up a half size and see if the shoe fits.

Special occasions require special clothes. It seems like every time I get pregnant there is a fancy dinner I need to attend or a wedding. Perhaps you found out you were invited to a wedding a few weeks before your due date—as the maid of honor. Yikes! Don't panic. They actually do make very nice dresses for special occasions, though usually for a pretty penny.

Bathing suits are also something that you might want to consider, no matter what time of year you are going to give birth. Water is such a comfort during pregnancy that I recommend it

▶ Sharing maternity clothes can work out very nicely, particularly if you have a friend or two who is about the same build. You can pass things back and forth with family members depending on the season and who is currently pregnant. This can be a very good way to get more bang for your maternity clothes buck. Be sure you label the clothes so you know who gets what back when you're done using them. I'd also suggest that you not exchange your favorite dress if you'd be beside yourself if something happened to it.

year-round when possible. That said, it is usually easier to swim in a bathing suit.

There are several options in maternity swimwear. One is to just buy a fun bikini and let it all hang out. This has become a very popular option recently. I see bikini-clad pregnant women at my pool all the time. If you don't want to bare the belly or share the stretch marks, that's okay too.

Consider a maternity bathing suit that has a skirt. This can be used well into postpartum too and hides any figure flaws you may worry about. The belly panels usually are very forgiving and can accommodate any size belly—big or small.

Size does matter. Maternity clothes are usually sized in a range from extra small (XS) to extra large (XL). However, some of the upper-end maternity stores try to project what they think you'll look like based on your size and boldly sell sized pregnancy clothes. So if you wore a size 12 before you were pregnant, you'd still choose a size 12 in their maternity wear.

Plus-sized women used to simply have to make do with whatever they could find. Now there are actually stores and lines of plus-sized maternity clothes, though these tend to be pricey.

No matter what your size, you're going to have to define your own style in pregnancy. Maternity clothes, normal clothes, bare midriff or not—it's your body. Remember you have to live in your skin and your clothes. Do what makes you feel comfortable and attractive.

Skin Care

Your skin, like every other part of your body, will undergo changes in pregnancy. For some women, these changes are pleasant, while other women complain about being covered with splotches and

ELSEWHERE ON THE WEB

▶ Belly Basics (www.belly-basics.com) has been working hard to put the fashion back in maternity fashion. Since their original invention of the Pregnancy Survival Kit, the whole maternity fashion world has been changed. The idea that a simple collection of clothes could take you comfortably and stylishly through an entire pregnancy is an amazing and simple concept that these guys do an awesome job with.

spots in pregnancy. To have healthy skin in pregnancy, consider the following:

- Use makeup that is safe in pregnancy.
- Wear sunscreen daily.
- Moisturize your body with lotion.
- If you have oily skin, use a gentle cleanser twice a day.
- Seek help from a dermatologist if problems get really bad or last beyond a few months postpartum.

Hopefully some of this is already incorporated into your morning beauty ritual anyway.

And before you think that I sit around and have facials every morning or wear tons of makeup, I don't. You still need to think of things like wearing sunscreen and moisturizer as maintaining your skin's beauty. You do not have to wear a lot of makeup to have healthy skin or to feel beautiful.

Are you glowing yet? We often describe a pregnant woman as glowing. The truth about your skin in pregnancy is that it is often not the glow you expected. Sometimes pregnancy is like being a teenager all over again. Unfortunately, acne can come with your new baby.

As in puberty, hormones are once again to blame for your acne in pregnancy. Usually your pregnant oily skin will clear up after the baby is born. Here are some helpful hints on dealing with acne in pregnancy:

- Hands off the acne—no poking or popping.
- Wash your face two times a day with a mild soap.
- Avoid makeup that is oil based.
- Never rub your skin, pat dry.

- Talk to your practitioner before using any over-the-counter acne products.
- Avoid Accutane in pregnancy.

The good news for some pregnant women who suffer from adult acne is that pregnancy can actually help clear up your skin. This does not apply to everyone, but doctors and midwives say that a good portion of those who have adult acne will see their face improve significantly.

While your face may tend to be oily, the rest of your body may actually suffer from dry skin. Trying to keep the rest of your body moisturized doesn't have to be a big long project. Simply choose a lotion that you like and remember to put it on daily. Putting it on after you get out of a bath or shower can help seal some of the moisture in your skin.

What's that dark line on your belly? Do not panic. It is called linea negra, which literally means black line. Normally you have a line in the same place but it's not noticeable.

The linea negra is a fairly common occurrence in pregnancy. It is caused by an increase in melanin in your pregnancy and is not harmful to you or your baby. The linea negra will generally go away within a few months after you have had your baby.

Despite what the old wives' tales say, the presence of the linea negra does not predict if you're carrying a boy or a girl. But don't be surprised if someone tells you that the line definitely means that there is a boy inside!

Does your face have splotchy spots? This is known as cholasma, or the mask of pregnancy. Cholasma usually appears on the forehead, cheeks, upper lip, and/or nose. Because of the location of the typical cholasma, it can look like a mask covering your face,

ELSEWHERE ON THE WEB

▶ Bras in pregnancy can be hard to figure out. I normally tell people to wear a good supportive bra during pregnancy and buy a nursing bra at the end. You need to know what types are available, how they are used, and most importantly how to find one that fits you. The Breastfeeding.com Web site has some great articles in their reading room, particularly on the subject of nursing bras:
www.breastfeeding.com/reading_room/nursing_bras/basics.html.

hence the name. Cholasma happens during pregnancy, when your body produces more melanin. This can cause certain areas of your body to become hyperpigmented or darker.

The American Academy of Dermatology (AAD) suggests that 70 percent of pregnant women will have some form of cholasma in pregnancy. Some women also experience this with some hormonal methods of birth control. Cholasma usually goes away without treatment after you have given birth or stopped the hormonal birth control.

Cholasma can occur or be made worse if your skin is exposed to the sun. To best deal with cholasma during pregnancy, your best bet is to use a broad-spectrum sunscreen, which covers both UVA and UVB rays, rated SPF 30 or higher. This is because cholasma can be made worse by exposure to the sun. This should become a part of your daily routine. Sunscreen should be applied throughout the day if you are outside.

Your best bet is to use makeup to blend skin tone differences if your skin is darker in some areas. This will not harm your skin or worsen the cholasma. A busy mom of two wrote me to say that having cholasma with her third pregnancy forced her to take sunscreen seriously, and she is now grateful to have had the extra reminder.

You might be tempted to try and get rid of the dark areas on your skin. But using chemical peels and lightening agents to try to reduce the dark areas of skin can be dangerous. Since the darker areas will most likely go away on their own, treatment is usually not indicated during pregnancy. If you do treat your skin with lightening agents, you run the risk of permanent discoloration of that area.

Makeup in pregnancy is not dangerous. Most women are able to keep their normal makeup routine. Keep an open mind when it comes to skin changes. You may need to make slight adjustments to the types of makeup you use or the way you wash your face to meet the needs of your pregnant skin.

If your eyes start to look tired or puffy in pregnancy from a lack of sleep or just general fatigue, consider using a cream concealer to cover up the dark circles. You can also cover the entire area with a translucent powder, either alone or on top of the concealer. Some products are available to help reduce puffiness, but you can also use a chilled face mask to produce similar results. These eye or face masks also work wonders for headaches.

Think about choosing new colors for your makeup. Do the ones you have now flatter your face and style? For an inexpensive makeover, go to your local mall and find a department store doing makeovers for free. You might find that you actually do like some new products and can test them out before you buy.

Hair Care

You have probably heard about the gorgeous locks that pregnancy supposedly produces. Well, for many women it is true. Pregnancy is a time of great hair. Bad hair days be gone!

Taking care of your hair in pregnancy should not be any different than it was before. You will still be able to wash, dry, and style it as you used to. It is safe to use shampoo, conditioner, and treatments made for normal hair. You should, however, watch any medicinal shampoos. Remember that your scalp can absorb chemicals, so it is always best to check with your practitioner before using medicated shampoos.

There are some things that pregnant women notice about their hair in pregnancy. The biggest change is that their hair appears to be thicker. This is because your body is so busy growing a baby that it does not have time to shed hair on a regular basis. (The sad part is that this hair is slated to go and seems to come out all at once in the postpartum period.)

BEFORE YOUR APPOINTMENT

▶ If you are concerned about the chemical ingredients in your makeup, be sure to make a list for your practitioner of the products that you use. If you are able to bring the specific ingredients, that is even better. Then your practitioner can see exactly what is in your cosmetic case. We often forget that our skin is a transport system that can carry chemicals throughout our bodies. Your skin doesn't know the difference between makeup and a medication patch.

Can I have a manicure while pregnant?

▶ Getting a manicure or pedicure can be a great way to relax and have nails to enjoy. I'd recommend avoiding acrylic nails and ensuring that your manicurist knows you're expecting. You may also wish to avoid some of the more noxious chemicals. Make sure you're in a well-ventilated room when getting a manicure or pedicure. You might even opt to skip the chemicals on your nails and go for a nice buff instead.

If you happen to be one of the few women whose hair seems to be thinning, try not to get upset. Sometimes if you have thin, brittle hair, the progesterone in pregnancy can add to this problem, making your hair more likely to break off. When your hair breaks off at the root it appears that you have thinning hair, but you really don't. This does not usually happen in every pregnancy. If it concerns you, talk to your midwife or doctor, as well as your hair stylist.

Look for easy hairstyles. While I'm not suggesting that you get caught up in the ponytail trap, there are easy ways to stay stylish and not spend a lot of time fussing with your hair.

If your hair is naturally straight, consider just adding some hair products to smooth it out while damp. You can let it dry naturally or blow it dry for a very smooth look. If you have curls or wish you had curls, consider some of the curling gels. You place these in damp hair and let air dry for a wave or more depending on your hair.

Coloring or dying your hair in pregnancy is relatively controversial. There have not been any human studies on the chemicals used in these products to unequivocally say they are safe for use in pregnancy. There have been some studies done on animals, but they were exposed to very high doses for long periods of time, not a very useful comparison. Most practitioners take the safe route. They generally recommend that you do not use these products during the first trimester.

Several women have written me saying that they also try to use more natural dyes, like henna. However, these natural products have not been tested for use in pregnancy either. You should probably also look for products that contain low or no ammonia in them for added safety.

While the hair on your head might be looking fine, you've got hair growing in other places too. The hair on your legs may also grow faster and coarser. A mother of three wrote to tell me that a good pair of tweezers and her razor were her best friends in pregnancy when it came to removing unwanted hair.

Basic beauty tips for pregnancy include these:

- Do a daily beauty routine that includes moisturizing and sunscreen.
- If you need it, exfoliate with a gentle cleanser once a week.
- When using makeup, highlight your most attractive features.
- Don't shy away from cover-up if you want it.
- Wear classic cuts that can do multiple styles easily.
- Choose styles that flatter your body and fashion sense.

Commemorating Your Belly

While you may not believe it now, you will miss your pregnant belly! It is so amazing how our bodies stretch and open to receive this new life. You put your hands on your belly and think, "I will never forget this feeling." The truth is that parenting and life happen, and slowly those memories do fade.

Commemorating your belly during pregnancy is something fun and unique to you and this pregnancy. It is also something that older children get a big kick out of helping you do.

Taking photos of your belly is a must. I love to see the pregnancy photos that women send me. Watching the belly grow is so neat! If you decide to do a series of photos, you may want to consider using the same location and or outfit. Some women have shown me pictures in which they wore a bikini or shorts so that you could really see the exposed abdomen growing as the pregnancy progressed. I would recommend choosing a specific time each week or month to take these photos. A good example of when to take the pictures might be the day you change weeks. So if you're due on a Sunday, you change weeks on a Sunday.

ELSEWHERE ON THE WEB

▶ Catherine Steinmann knows a thing or two about pregnancy portraits. She has been doing them for decades. Her specialty is the pregnant nude. Though the word "nude" is used, these artsy photos involve lots of materials and fabrics to produce a very attractive portrait of pregnancy. Steinmann's work includes two volumes of her photographic works on pregnancy and others. Check out her Web site: www.about pregnancyphoto.com.

Professional photographers are also doing many more maternity portraits. These can be done alone or with your partner or children. To find someone who does these types of portraits, just search the Web for family portrait photographers in your area.

Painting your belly is simple. You can do this at any point in your pregnancy. Some moms write to say they do this on a monthly basis. One mom even said that was how she announced her pregnancy. She painted blue and pink hearts on her abdomen and waited for her husband to notice.

You can use any kind of nontoxic paint for belly painting. Poster paints are the least expensive, though paints made for makeup or the stage are easier on the skin. This is particularly noteworthy if you intend to wear the paint for long periods of time.

What you draw or paint is personal. Have fun and be creative. People have sent pictures for the belly gallery of their bellies painted as basketballs or pumpkins. This can also be a great costume for Halloween or other events.

Here's what you will need to paint your pregnant belly:

- Paint
- Paint brushes, different sizes
- Drop cloth or towel to catch spills
- Camera to record the event

Some businesses specialize in pregnancy art. Check the Web or phone book to find someone locally. Try going to a local art school or studio to see if someone is interested in experimenting!

Belly casting is another popular way to record your belly. This is done by making a plaster mold of your abdomen. You can also choose to do your torso in addition to your abdomen. How much you choose to encase in plaster is up to you. You can purchase kits to do the belly casting. These make great shower gifts. Or you can assemble the items yourself. Here's what you need to do a belly cast:

- Plaster-impregnated gauze strips
- Petroleum jelly (or unpetroleum jelly)
- Plastic wrap
- Drop cloth
- Bowl of hot water
- Scissors

You will start by cutting the gauze into long (twelve-inch), medium (six-inch), and short (two- to three-inch) strips. Cover any part of your body you are going to cast with the petroleum jelly. The jelly is used to help the cast come off once it is completed. Then cover any hair, particularly your pubic hair, with the plastic wrap. The plastic wrap sticks to the jelly for ease in keeping it on.

Strike a pose while sitting on a chair or stool over the drop cloth and have your husband start dipping the longer strips of the gauze in the water to activate the plaster. He will cover the entire area you intend to cast with the wet strips of gauze. You will want to do several layers to make the finished product thick. Use the smaller strips to help get curves, particularly around your belly button or breasts. These help with details.

When you're done putting the plaster strips on the cast, you need to tap around the cast to see if it is hard. You can usually feel it start to harden even before you get to the top layers. When it is hard, just slide the cast off and rest it on a towel where it can dry.

Once dry, the cast can become many things. Some families choose to paint it and use it as a decoration. These do look great, painted or unpainted, as baby shower decorations.

TOOLS YOU NEED

▶ Francine Krause has been doing belly casts, or belly masks, as she calls them, for a very long time. She has a gorgeous collection of belly casts in her gallery as well as a belly casting kit and do-it-yourself video. Included in her kit are all the products you need to make the cast and instructions to make, finish, and mount the kit. You can find her on the Web at www.bellymask.com.

Get Linked

Pregnancy doesn't have to be a time to be ugly. More and more women feel beautiful in pregnancy. There is no reason you shouldn't feel that way, too. Wear fun clothes, enjoy your new body, and always do something to celebrate your belly!

MATERNITY CLOTHES

If you're interested in the latest fashions in pregnancy and what kind of clothes there are to buy, look no further. Included are tips on when to wear maternity clothes, buying maternity clothes, spending less and loving them more, bathing suits, and much more.

 http://about.com/pregnancy/maternityclothes

BODY PIERCINGS AND TATTOOS

Interested in seeing what happens to body piercings and tattoos in pregnancy? Check out this photo gallery.

 http://about.com/pregnancy/piercingtattoo

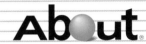

Chapter 7

The Fun Stuff

What Do Babies Really Need?

Having a baby seems to induce a shopping frenzy in many people. A positive pregnancy test will send someone shopping faster than any other medical test known to man. Think about it—what did you buy when you found out you were expecting?

While I will give you plenty of lists of products in this chapter, I have to start by telling you that the most important thing your baby needs is you. Your baby will need to be held, changed, and fed. These are the most important things you need for your baby. Of course, there are a few basics that everyone needs from day one:

- ○ A couple of outfits
- ○ Diapers
- ○ Car seat

Beyond that everything else is optional, though totally fun to shop for!

Going beyond the basics for baby is what most people choose to do. More and more people are buying more and more stuff for babies. It is very hard not to go overboard when buying that adorable baby-style stuff. I mean, they have such cute prints and the fabrics are so soft. Who could resist?

Try to resist the urge to buy too much stuff. Do keep in mind it is one tiny little baby. And you have to find space for all of that stuff. So many moms write me to say that they fell into the trap of having to have every piece of equipment, only to figure out that their baby hated the swing or the bouncy chair.

For that reason, I'd highly recommend that you keep your spending to a minimum until after your baby is born. Let her test out someone else's bouncy chair before buying one for your house and grandma's house. You might find she hates it. Which means you could be stuck with a piece of furniture you never use.

Most parents buy more than the minimum. A more realistic list of items for baby would include:

- Co-sleeper or bassinet
- Car seat (at least one, maybe two depending on car situation)
- Changing table
- Baby sling or carrier
- Rocking chair or glider
- Dresser
- Diaper pail
- Diapers (cloth or disposable—a dozen cloth, with covers, or several dozen disposables)
- Clothes (indoor and outdoor)
  - 8 onesies (long or short sleeve depending on the season)
  - 2 hats
  - 2 outfits (for dressing up or pictures)

- I sweater
- 3 blankets
- 3 sleepers (weight depends on season and where baby is sleeping)
- Swing
- Baby bath tub
- Hooded towels (two)
- Bouncy seat
- Baby monitor (only if you're away from baby)
- High chair (not usually needed immediately)
- Toys (a couple, you can add on later)
- Books (a couple of your favorites to read to baby from birth)

It can be a daunting task to figure out what pieces really work for you and what don't. My best advice is to talk to other new parents. Don't get swayed by advertising. Find out what other people who are really using these products are saying.

Buying for baby can be costly. You can save your budget if you plan and shop well. You may be able to borrow some bigger-ticket items or buy them used. A high chair is a good example of something that works well used. A bit of soapy water and bleach and you've got a great new-to-you high chair, for probably a third of the cost of a brand-new one.

The same idea works for many baby items. Try looking for consignment or secondhand stores that specialize in maternity clothes and baby products. They are usually very good places to look for bargains. You might also find that certain child-related organizations have regular yard sales. Many Mothers of Twins Clubs do offer clothing and equipment sales yearly. These are always good places to find gently used items.

ELSEWHERE ON THE WEB

▶ Consumer Reports (www.consumerreports.org) has built its reputation on good-quality safety reviews. The book *Consumer Reports Best Baby Products* is no exception. One of the things that I really like about the site is the handy information on safety recalls. Epinions (www.epinions.com) is another great site with a large selection of information about baby products from strollers to high chairs and more. It is a fabulous way to figure out how the products you are looking at really perform. It also gives you a chance to let others know your thoughts on a product.

When should I begin buying baby things?

▶ The answer to this question varies widely. Some parents choose to hold off purchasing baby items until the very last minute for superstitious reasons or fear that something may happen to their baby. Others take the approach that they need to be prepared for baby while they have the time and/or money. Sometimes purchases are made on a whim, during a big sale. It's normal to start thinking about your purchases soon, but when you choose to actually make them is totally up to you and your pocketbook.

When buying or borrowing used baby equipment, the number-one thing to remember is safety. How old is a crib you're looking at? Does it have lead paint? Are the slats 2 3/8 inches or more apart? Does this item meet current safety standards? The only thing I insist on buying for every child is a car seat. With a used car seat you can never be sure if it was in a previous wreck or if it meets the latest standards. However, not everyone agrees with me on that issue.

And don't hesitate to ask your friends or relatives to share big items. You might find that a hand-me-down is perfect for your needs. This is also a good idea for you to consider when a relative in your family is pregnant—offer some of your stash! This is where so many of my readers say they found the best products for their babies.

Some items you use only for a brief period of time and then they are no longer useful. You need to decide if you can get the item combined with another in a multi-use product. A good example of this would be the bassinet features that fit inside most portable play yards. Some even come with changing areas as well.

Do you need a baby crib?   This question might be more difficult to answer than it appears on the surface. A crib is a place where your baby sleeps. Sounds obvious, right?

Lots of mothers and fathers have written to say that they had once assumed that a crib was the most important piece of baby equipment they needed. What some of these parents found was that a crib was most useful for holding baby clothes and toys. They found that their baby, for one reason or another, rarely slept in the crib. This was particularly true in the first few months.

In the early months, babies sleep best near their parents. For some mothers and fathers this is in a cradle, a bassinet or a basket right next to their bed or in their room. While these parents may have received flack from other family members, the American Academy of Pediatrics (AAP) now backs them up. In a recent statement, the AAP has said that babies should sleep in close proximity to their parents.

Some parents decide that the family bed or co-sleeping is what works for their family. The family bed has proponents and detractors. As with any parenting options, do your homework and figure out what works for you.

Co-sleeping can be a safe and viable option for many families. Be sure to follow certain safety rules, including these:

- Never sleep with a baby when you have been drinking or taking medication.
- Do not use fluffy blankets or large pillows near baby.
- Your mattress should be firm.
- Do not co-sleep on a couch, water bed, or other soft surface.
- Never leave your baby alone in your bed, even while sleeping.
- Do not wear night clothes with strings or ribbons.
- Use mesh rails if your bed is off the floor.
- If you are overweight, co-sleeping may not be safe.

If you choose to use a crib, there are also safety guidelines that go along with that purchase:

- Slats should be no further apart than 2 3/8 inches.
- Mattress should be firm and tight-fitting. You should be able to get no more than two fingers between the crib and the mattress.
- Avoid cutouts in the wood of the foot or headboard.
- Corner posts should be no more than 1/16 of an inch high, unless they are canopy height.

ELSEWHERE ON THE WEB

▶ Baby products can be dangerous. Look for well-known brands with good safety records and few recalls. Check out the Baby Products site on About.com: http://babyproducts.about.com. The U.S. Consumer Product Safety Commission (www.cpsc.gov) also has a wealth of resources as you're trying to stock your baby's nursery or your home. You can sign up for e-mails on the latest recalls, view safety tips for every room in your house, and much more.

- Never use bumper pads, comforters, pillows, or stuffed animals in your baby's crib.

There are many options available when purchasing a crib. For example, if you don't have a lot of space, you may consider a mini-crib or a portable mesh crib. Perhaps you'd like to buy a crib that will last you a lot longer than a year or two. This can be done by getting a crib that converts to a toddler bed. There are also cribs that can be converted to an adult size. The only drawback there is that you may outgrow the style by then.

Decorating Your Nursery

Once you have figured out where your baby will be, then you can find the perfect ideas for the room. Some mothers-to-be do the room early on so that they can be sure to have the energy. Others find that having the nursery to decorate helped them connect with their baby as well as their spouse, giving them a joint project to work on.

The first step to decorating your nursery is to map out the room. You don't have to have a degree in design to sit down with a pencil and paper and draw some ideas of ways to lay out the room. Here are some basics to remember when planning your baby's nursery:

- Avoid putting the crib in any part of the room that gets direct sunlight during the day or illumination from outside at night.
- Build in storage space. If you don't have a closet, consider a way to add more storage.
- Be sure to have a place for grown-ups in your plan.
- Don't overcrowd the room.

ELSEWHERE ON THE WEB

▶ Co-sleeping is done by many families, though they may be fearful to admit it. Co-sleeping is safe when certain standards are followed. William Sears, M.D., and Martha Sears, R.N., are well known for their research and study of co-sleeping, in addition to their personal experience with co-sleeping. Their Web site has a resource center designed for questions about the practice of co-sleeping and the family bed, at www.askdrsears.com.

Once you have the room drawn up with your basic ideas, then you can start planning the actual pieces to go in the room. Think about your needs for that room. What do you envision doing there? Do you anticipate changing the baby there? Feeding the baby? This will help you decide what you need for the room.

Painting the room can add a lot of color. If you choose to not use wallpaper or permanent decorations over the paint, the room can easily be revitalized as your child grows. Color choice is personal. Some families choose to stick with calm shades, while others go for primary colors. It's totally up to you.

Floor covering is something you may not have given a lot of thought to prior to having a baby. My advice is to get rid of the wall-to-wall carpeting. Not only is it a huge allergy issue, but it is a bear to clean. Hardwood or laminate floors are much easier with a little one. Baby messes wipe up quickly, and you can just dust the floors to keep them clean.

You can still decorate even if you don't have a nursery.
Not everyone has the room to have a separate nursery. You may have a special area set aside in your room for the baby and all the baby things. Perhaps your older child will be sharing a room with the new baby. These are all real possibilities when preparing for a new baby, but don't let them deter you from a bit of decorating.

If the baby will be joining you in your room, try to have a small area that can be dedicated to baby things. At the same time, keep in mind no matter how much space you allocate for baby stuff, it winds up taking over your house. In the space you have, are there decorations already up that you can remove easily? If not, don't sweat it. Your baby doesn't know the difference between an expensive baby toy and the framed poster of a famous artist. The point is to stimulate the brain.

If you have a baby crib, consider a theme (bears, for example). You can buy matching sheets, similar colors for other items in the area, and perhaps a comforter to match. (Use this as a wall decoration because it is not appropriate in a crib with your baby.)

If your baby will be sharing a room with a sibling, involve your older child in the decorating process. This will help your older child feel more a part of the process and less like the baby is taking over his room. You might have him help pick a color from a handful of your finalists, as long as you're truly ready to go with that choice.

Sharing a room with you or with siblings is not a bad thing. There is something to be said for learning to share at such an early age. You also do not need to give up the fun of decorating a space for your new arrival, even in the room-sharing situation.

Choosing Baby Names

Choosing a name for your baby is special. It should be a time of fun, but many women tell me horror stories about trying to name their babies. Some of the stories involve nightmare family relations and people trying to dictate what the baby should be named. Others are simply stories of not being able to find a name they like—or worse, a name that can be agreed upon.

There is not just one way to pick a baby name, though the fights and tears that can sometimes go along with naming a baby should be avoided. I find that these fights come from various places.

Don't pick names to annoy one another.   I admit I'm guilty of this one. When my husband refuses to play the baby-naming game, I get mad and start choosing names I know make him cringe. It serves no purpose except to make him shut down further. So I do not advise this tactic.

You both need to genuinely like people you are naming after. It is simply not fair to choose a name you like, all the while knowing your other half hates it for whatever reason. Sometimes this boils down to not using a name you like because of the person associated with the name.

You wouldn't want to name your baby after his ex-girlfriend, even if you loved the name. Perhaps your husband has suggested the name of an old teacher, and all you can remember is that he gave you detention. It is possible to like a name and still not be able to use it.

There is no perfect time to start looking at names. One mom-to-be told me that she and her husband decided on names for their children on their second date. I had to laugh because my baby-naming style has changed so much in just the last few years I can't imagine having chosen names years in advance. Apparently, however, this technique works for quite a few couples.

You may want to get started early if you think there are going to be large differences of opinion. This will give you more time so that you don't feel like the due date is staring you down. Even if you aren't ready to start sharing your ideas together as a couple, consider leafing through some name books, just to have an idea of some names you might consider.

I like to read through names and then come up with lists. This means I get to read baby names and pretend to pick names all day long, without annoying my husband. It turns out that my husband—and there are many like him—doesn't like to think of names too soon. He wants to lay eyes on the baby. He prefers not to sit around and go through name after name to get there.

Try this exercise. Make a list of your top five or ten names for girls and boys, and have your partner do the same. Then trade lists. You each can cross off a certain number of names, no questions

ELSEWHERE ON THE WEB

▶ The Name Voyager at the Baby Name Wizard site (www.babynamewizard.com) is so much fun! I was totally prepared to be underwhelmed by yet another baby name site, but this one is different. You plug in a name or the start of a name and see a graphical representation of how popular that name has been over the past hundred years. It is also in pink or blue so you can see those gender names. My husband even relented and looked at it. He had a lot of fun looking around too. This is absolutely a dad-friendly site.

asked. You might find yourself left with some names you can agree upon, like Clare versus Clara.

Once you have made these lists, start the discussion. Maybe you weren't lucky enough to get the same names or even similar names. But maybe you can tell that you both like exotic names, like Lilah, Hadar, Sabine, or Aviyah. Try to follow that genre of name until you can find one you both agree on.

What should you look for in a name?   Names are personal choices, so try not to get bullied by anyone. One dad wrote me to say that he was offered a large sum of money if he named the baby after a certain relative. He wanted my advice on convincing his wife to use that name. I just couldn't do it.

Here are some ideas of what to look for in a name:

- You both like the name.
- There aren't any nicknames you dislike associated with it (such as "Dick" for Richard)
- The initials aren't potentially embarrassing (as with "April Samantha Stivers").
- The name doesn't belong to someone your child might not like to be named after.

There are only a couple of other things to think about when naming your baby. These may not be deal breakers, but they do deserve consideration:

- Is it pronounceable?
- Is it easily spelled?
- Does the name follow your religious or cultural beliefs?

- Did you choose a name that meant something to you or your family?
- Does the name have a pleasant meaning?

Do you like popular names?   Every year the Social Security Administration publishes a list of the most popular baby names. It is definitely a fun thing to keep an eye on, but what does it mean to you as an expectant parent? This list can be handy if you want to avoid the superpopular names so your daughter isn't the third Amanda in her class.

Does finding out the sex make your list shorter?   It might! If you choose to find out whether you're carrying a girl or a boy, you might only have to look for half the names. Though more than one mom has told me that they were surprised when the baby was born and they didn't have a name for a baby of that particular gender.

My advice? Have a couple of backup names. Even if you got the boy you were expecting, you might look at him and just know that he is not the Jackson that you thought he would be. He might very obviously be a Carter or a Teddy or a Reese.

Don't panic if the baby is here and you don't have a name yet.   You might get pressured into having a name immediately, but most states give you plenty of time to make your choice. It merely holds up paperwork if you don't have the name by the time you leave the hospital or birth center. To find out what the rules are where you live, call your state's Department of Vital Statistics.

In the end, you will find a name. It will hopefully be a name you both love and that makes you smile when you look at your child. I always remind myself, too, that the baby can change it later if he or she really hates it.

TOOLS YOU NEED

▶ Everyone needs a good baby-name book. There are plenty to choose from. Decide what you want in a baby-name book. Do you want every name you could ever imagine? Perhaps you want to narrow it down to a specific genre? Ask around about baby-name books others enjoy and use frequently. Then look through them yourself at the bookstore or online. You'll be spending a lot of time with the book.

The Baby Shower: Throwing a Perfect Party

Everyone loves to celebrate a new baby! Okay, almost everyone. The trick to throwing a great baby shower is to remember to keep it positive, fun, and not terribly goofy.

There are a few things you have to have in order to throw a great baby shower:

○ Theme
○ Invitations
○ Decorations
○ Food
○ Games
○ Gifts

Keeping these six things in mind, you can put together a very nice baby shower on any budget. It is also important to keep the mother-to-be in mind. If you're trying to make a decision about a shower and you can't or don't want to involve the mother, ask yourself how she would feel about whatever it is you're deciding on.

Baby shower themes usually set the tone for the party.

A theme should be something that the mother-to-be is interested in, like a nursery theme to match her nursery. Some families choose a theme based on the gender of the baby or a pattern they saw in the party store. There isn't a right or wrong answer here.

Whatever theme you do choose will help you pick decorations, plates, gifts, and so on. But don't get stressed out by picking a theme. It can be something as simple as a color combination or as extravagant as specific pattern.

Shower invitations are the face of your shower. The invitation will tell your guests everything they need to know about your shower. It should have the following information at a minimum:

- The name of the mother being showered
- The day and date of the shower
- The time of the shower
- The location of the shower
- How to RSVP
- Any special information needed

Anything beyond the above is considered additional. You might include a map, particularly if your guests do not know where they are going. Other party hostesses choose include information on shower festivities that require outside help, like you bringing a picture of yourself as a baby.

Invitation etiquette can be difficult. If you're in charge of sending out the invitations, you might wonder whether it's appropriate to list where the mother-to-be is registered. I think most people appreciate the notice. Every store imaginable has a baby gift registry, and this is handy information for your guests to have in advance. If it bothers you, simply leave it out and tell any guests who ask.

Depending on how far guests have to travel, you will want to send the invitations out with plenty of advance warning. For small, close-knit families or communities, two weeks is plenty of time.

You should have one central place for RSVP collection so you can get a more accurate head count. Whenever I am throwing a party, I try to keep a list of the guests near the phone. Then when people call me to say yes or no, I can mark it down right away. This method is also helpful if other people answer your phone, like your husband or children.

ELSEWHERE ON THE WEB

▶ While baby shower invitations used to be handwritten, now you'll find invitations that are sent via e-mail. I think it's really great and saves a lot of anxiety about keeping everyone straight if you use a free program like Evite (www.evite.com). They actually have several invitation styles to choose from, and you get to use your own wording. Not to mention the glorious fact that your guests can RSVP online!

Decorations add to the atmosphere. A little bit can go a long way in making your party area seem warm and inviting. You can do simple balloons in certain colors, small table decorations, or even a flower bouquet.

Baby showers are generally not huge on decorations. The biggest bash I've seen involved some balloons, streamers, a sign on the lawn, and a cute poster display of all the shower attendees as babies. You can have as much or as little as you see fit, but do discuss your ideas with the hostess, if possible.

Your food will likely be determined by the time of day. How you plan for food should be based on the time of day you selected for the shower. Most baby showers are either lunch affairs or mid-afternoon functions with snacks.

If you are offering a lunch menu it is still usually a light lunch of sandwiches, fruit or pasta salad, and cake for dessert. You may also offer other types of food depending on what you feel comfortable doing.

Drinks can be soft drinks and water, though some showers do different drinks. I personally love punch, and a baby shower is a great excuse to have it. Punch can be very simple, and yet looks like you worked very hard. Here is my favorite recipe:

- 1 gallon rainbow sherbet
- 4 liters lemon-lime soda, such as Sprite

Put the rainbow sherbet in a bowl and pour the Sprite over it. This makes a beautiful and delicious punch. For quick decorations, consider adding frozen fruit to float in the punch. I'd avoid the frozen blueberries as they may be a choking hazard.

Dessert at a baby shower is typically a cake. Some cakes are very creative and done in the form of a sleeping baby. They might be decorated with a picture of the mother and/or father-to-be as babies. Many are simply sheet cakes with warm welcoming wishes written in pink or blue.

You might consider setting out small snacks around the sitting area. You can do nuts and small candies like M&Ms, which can be purchased in pinks or blues. You could also do specialty candies wrapped with sayings like "It's a boy!"

Baby shower games are not to be dreaded.   Still, "dread" is a word you will often hear associated with baby shower games, some of which are often quite goofy and even out of control in some situations. When choosing the games that will make your baby shower fun, keep a few things in mind:

- Who are your guests?
- How much time and preparation will each game will take?
- What will the mother-to-be prefer?

The final decision should always lie in what the guest of honor would like the most. If she's a fun-lovin' gal who would think that tasting baby food would be cool, go for it! But if the mother-to-be is a bit more prim and proper, you'd be better off sticking with games that are a bit more in line with her way of thinking.

Most shower hostesses give small gifts for those that win games. These gifts need not be anything big or fancy. Some common items are small stationery sets, candles, or photo frames.

Gifts are often the focus of baby showers.   Whether this is intentional or not, it does happen. Figure out how the mother-to-be feels about this type of shower. Some people are embarrassed to open gifts in front of others, particularly with all the oohing and ahhing over the cute baby outfits. If she doesn't mind,

WHAT'S HOT

▶ Reusable decorations are always a big hit. There are adorable diaper cakes made of diapers (cloth or disposables) and filled with baby toys and necessities like baby washcloths, socks, lotion, etc. They are made to use as decorations, but then when the shower is over you can open them up and use each of the items for baby.

▸ A quick shower game that also helps out the mother-to-be is to have everyone self-address an envelope provided by the hostess. Then she is given these with a pack of thank you notes. This allows her to not have to deal with addressing envelopes. To make it a game, the envelopes are collected in a bag or basket. The mother-to-be then draws an envelope out of the container and that person is given a small prize.

go for it, but if she does, perhaps consider letting her open the presents alone later.

While baby gift registries are quite popular, not everyone will shop off these registries. Some people have standard shower gifts they give at every baby shower. This is a good thing; it provides the parents-to-be with gifts they may not have thought about registering for, particularly if they are new parents. I personally try to always give useful items. One thing I like to do is to fill up a baby bathtub or diaper pail with small useful items like infant nail clippers, infant medicine packs, socks, and onesies.

Couples showers are becoming more popular. You may have heard of people doing this themselves. It can be a lot of fun for everyone. Dads don't get enough recognition and if your husband is game, I'd recommend you go for it.

That said, a couple's shower is usually much different than a regular baby shower. The emphasis is usually much less on baby games and more on the get-together. There are very few strictly baby themed couple showers. I'd recommend that you think about planning a potluck meal or a restaurant shower.

Blessingways

Blessingways are spiritual gatherings. These are usually woman-centered events that are done in addition to or in place of the traditional baby shower. The focus of a blessingway is more on the mother-to-be and her journey to motherhood.

The goal of a blessingway is to boost the mother-to-be. She should feel supported and cared for both during and after the ceremony. This is done by a series of caring events done during the Blessingway. Most people who hold a blessingway choose a couple of activities, such as these:

- Creation of a necklace for use in labor or nursing
- Prayer flags
- Matrilineal introductions (for example: I am Robin, daughter of Carol, granddaughter of Carolyn, and great granddaughter of Amanda.)
- Smudging of the space (ceremonious spiritual cleansing by burning sage)
- Singing
- Sharing a meal
- Making a belly cast

Typically gifts are given, particularly gifts like car seats and baby clothes. If the guests bring anything, it is usually things like beads for a necklace to be made for the expectant mother or candles for her to use in labor. There may also be a gift book made of positive birth and parenting affirmations.

Blessingways are very special ceremonies. I cannot begin to tell you how special I felt when my friends held one for me during my twin pregnancy. It really helped carry me through the end of a rough time knowing I had them on my side. Other women have also written me with glowing reports of the feeling of love and support they received from being blessed like this.

TOOLS YOU NEED

▶ *Blessingways: A Guide to Mother-Centered Baby Showers,* by Shari Maser, is the ultimate resource for planning a blessingway. It has ideas for invitations, food, songs, and ceremonial happenings. This book is a must-have if you decide to do a blessingway.

Get Linked

Baby names, nurseries, and baby showers are fun parts of pregnancy. No matter how much you know, there is still a lot to learn about picking furniture, baby names, and everything else your baby will need.

BABY PRODUCTS

Looking for information on the best baby products available? I can help you steer clear of products that aren't worth your time or money as well as help you find the perfect baby shower gift.

 http://about.com/pregnancy/babyproducts

BABY NAMES

Here you'll find articles on how to find the best name for your baby, including a name dictionary, how to name twins, and debates on gender names.

 http://about.com/pregnancy/babynames

BABY SHOWERS

Everyone loves a great party, and baby showers are the greatest! If you are looking for games, decorations, the perfect present, or anything related to baby showers, come see the collection of articles on everything from baby shower etiquette to our e-mail course on planning the perfect party.

 http://about.com/pregnancy/babyshowers

BLESSINGWAYS

This spiritual and soulful alternative to a typical baby shower is perfect for any mother-to-be who needs to feel love and support from her friends and family.

 http://about.com/pregnancy/blessingway

Chapter 8

Complications in Pregnancy

When to Call the Practitioner

One of your biggest fears in pregnancy is probably that something will go wrong. The good news is that for most women, this is simply a fear and not a fact. That does not stop you from being worried. It is nice to know that you have someone to call and talk to about your questions.

Most of us start with our friends or family when we have questions. Perhaps you have sent me an e-mail asking me your question, but the best person to answer most of your questions is your practitioner. He knows you, your baby, your pregnancy, and your health history best. That's not to say that the advice you get from others is not valuable; it's just not as medically precise as it could be.

There is nothing as intimidating as calling your doctor or midwife's office when you are scared or nervous and encountering a phone bank with a ton of numbered options. Only you know whether or not you should call. My advice is that if you think you

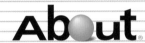

should call, then call. Some helpful guidelines are to call if you have any of the following symptoms:

- Bleeding
- Pain
- Contractions prior to 37 weeks of pregnancy
- Gush of fluid from your vagina
- Sudden severe headache
- Swelling
- Change in fetal movement questions
- Questions that cannot wait until your next appointment

When you call, you need to have certain information handy to make the phone call go as smoothly as possible. The ideal thing to do is to carry this information with you at all times so it is quickly ready in an emergency. If you don't have it together, call your practitioner anyway, as there will be time to gather it as needed later. Here are the items you need to include:

- Your name
- Due date
- First day of your last menstrual period
- Symptoms you are experiencing (pain, bleeding, fluid, temperature, etc.)
- How long you've been having these symptoms
- Name of your doctor or midwife
- Hospital closest to you
- Pharmacy name and number

If you call after regular business hours or during a lunch break, your call may be routed to an answering service or answering machine. The answering service will either call the practitioner or leave a message, depending on why you say you are calling. If they tell you it will be awhile before you get a call back, you have the right to ask for another doctor or midwife in the call schedule or to go to the emergency room. Do not wait at home in a severe emergency like suspected preterm labor, bleeding, or pain.

After you have called the answering service, your practitioner will usually call you back within a few minutes. If you have not received a call within about five or ten minutes, call the answering service again. They can tell you how to proceed.

If you call your midwife or doctor during business hours, you may be routed to the nurse or a physician's assistant for help. This person can help you determine if you should come to the office immediately, be met at the emergency room, or simply keep your next appointment. If it is not an emergency, you may have to wait until the end of the day to speak to your practitioner.

Problems with Mom

Problems are not what you want to experience in your pregnancy. However, sometimes they do occur. The hardest thing is usually separating what is a problem for you and what is a problem for your baby, as many of the things that might bother you could ultimately bother your baby as well.

Rh factor is a component of your blood type.
Early in pregnancy, when you have a lot of blood work done, your practitioner will check your blood type (A, B, O, AB) as well as your Rh factor (either positive or negative).

If either you or your partner is Rh positive, you have the possibility of having a baby who is Rh positive. Problems arise if the baby is positive and you are negative. You could accidentally be exposed to the baby's blood (most likely during birth or medical procedures like an amniocentesis, cesarean section, or miscarriage). This is not

ASK YOUR GUIDE

I often worry about bothering my practitioner for what seems like small questions or concerns. What can I do?

▶ I have talked to so many women who are worried about being a bother when calling the office. I will tell you what I tell them: You are paying for the services of your doctor or midwife. Of course, you are paying for her time to answer appropriate questions at an appropriate time. You shouldn't call to schedule an appointment at 8 P.M., nor page the practitioner on call with a routine question in the middle of the night. As long as you're respectful, she should be happy to help you.

a problem with your first pregnancy. It is potentially a problem in subsequent pregnancies if you have been exposed and your body has created antibodies. If this happens, your body believes that the new pregnancy is a foreign substance and tries to protect you by attacking the baby. This can lead to prematurity or stillbirth. To prevent that from happening, an Rh-negative woman gets a shot of Rhogam late in pregnancy and again at birth.

Anemia is routinely tested for in pregnancy. You are most likely to become anemic toward the end of your pregnancy. Your body will expand its blood volume by 50 percent near the second half of pregnancy, and your body will need more iron to make more hemoglobin to oxygenate that blood. Your baby and placenta will also have more needs.

Prevention of anemia is always the best option. The easiest way to do that is to eat a diet rich in iron. This can include beans, tofu, dark-green leafy vegetables, broccoli, whole-grain breads and pastas, raisins, pumpkin, sweet potatoes, and iron-fortified cereals. You do not need to eat meat to get the recommended amounts of iron, though red meat and dark-meat chicken are good sources.

The good news is that even if you are mildly anemic, your baby is not likely to have any problems. Your body supplies your baby's needs first. However, severe anemia or first-trimester anemia can lead to an increased risk of preterm labor.

Some symptoms of anemia include the following:

- Being overly tired
- Pale skin
- Palpitations
- Feeling of weakness
- Dizzy spells or fainting
- Getting winded easily

Iron-deficiency anemia can be fairly common in pregnancy, especially if you are carrying multiple babies, have had two pregnancies relatively close together, or are having problems with nutrition due to severe nausea and vomiting.

The treatment for your anemia will depend on the type you have.

Supplementation is the most common form of treatment, particularly for iron-deficiency anemia. While most prenatal vitamins have some amount of supplement, you will likely need more if you are already suffering from anemia.

The Centers for Disease Control (CDC) recommend that pregnant women get about 30 mg of elemental iron a day to prevent anemia. If you are already anemic, you will require more. Ferrous sulfate is the supplement most often found in vitamins. A supplement of 325 mg of ferrous sulfate will provide you with about 60 mg of elemental iron.

The trickiest part of iron supplementation is getting your body to absorb the iron. It's best to avoid caffeine and calcium while taking your iron supplement. Calcium can be found in some vitamins, antacids, and in products like milk and dairy. Allow as much time as possible between eating these things and taking your iron supplement.

Taking your iron on an empty stomach with orange juice (or another food high in vitamin C) can also help absorption. Just be sure that your orange juice is not the type that is filled with calcium. You can also eat your iron-rich foods. Cooking with cast iron also helps increase your absorption of iron.

The biggest problem visitors to my site complain about is the constipation and stomach ills from supplementation. I recommend increasing your fiber intake if you have to take supplemental iron. The extra fiber can be in any form, like adding prunes or dates to your diet; some women like to add more vegetables. I've also found that the liquid supplements seem to work better for some women.

There are so many infections that are possible to contract in pregnancy. How can I educate myself?

▶ Staying up to date on each and every infection can be difficult. Luckily, MedlinePlus (www.nlm .nih.gov/medlineplus/ infectionsandpregnancy .html) lists the most common infections, infor- mation on treatment, com- plications, and cures. This includes information on bacterial vaginosis, rubella, listeria, cytomegalovirus (CMV), and many others.

Infections during pregnancy can cause complications. Infections can be viral or bacterial. In fact, certain types of infection can cause a large portion of the preterm labor cases. This is why knowing about infections can be a very important part of preg- nancy health.

Be sure to talk to your midwife or doctor about different signs and symptoms that you should report to them. Remember that infections can be systemic or localized. Here are some things to keep in mind about infection in pregnancy:

- Good hygiene goes a long way, so wash your hands and your food well and often.
- Avoid small children with contagious diseases like chicken pox.
- Ensure that your immunizations are up to date, preferably before you get pregnant.
- Consider whether you need additional vaccines, like a flu shot.
- Avoid travel to high-infection-risk areas.

Group B strep goes by many names. You may hear it dis- cussed as GBS, beta strep, etc. Group B strep occurs in about 25 percent of all pregnant women. It is not a sexually transmitted disease and it will not harm you or your partner. In fact, it is only a potential problem for your baby in a certain set of circumstances.

Most practitioners routinely screen every pregnant woman in their care between thirty-five and thirty-seven weeks of preg- nancy. This screening is done by taking a vaginal and rectal swab to check for the group B strep bacteria. If the test is negative, nothing further happens.

If the test is positive, you will receive intravenous (IV) antibiot- ics during labor. Though chances are slim that your baby would be positive if you received these antibiotics, your baby will be monitored after birth just in case.

If you do not know your group B strep status when you go into labor, you will only be treated if you run a fever in labor, your water is broken for a prolonged period of time (usually more than eighteen hours), you have had a previous baby who had group B strep, or you are in preterm labor.

Group B strep does not affect breastfeeding in any manner. You should continue to breastfeed your baby as planned. Nor does group B strep necessitate a cesarean birth.

Thyroid disease is common in women. Whether you've been diagnosed as hypothyroid or hyperthyroid, pregnancy is a time when your hormones run wild. It is very important that you see your doctor or midwife immediately, as the vast majority of women with thyroid disease require more thyroid replacement hormone in pregnancy.

Screening for thyroid disorders in pregnancy is not yet universal. But the risks of thyroid disease to the baby include preterm labor, miscarriage, and lowered IQ. This makes it very important to be screened. If your practitioner does not suggest this screening blood test, you have the right to request it.

If you are diagnosed with thyroid disease, you will need to have your blood drawn periodically. This will continue throughout pregnancy and into the postpartum time period. Most women will need an increase in their medications, some by as much as 50 percent.

Since pregnancy and postpartum are such hormonal events, it is a time when many women are diagnosed with thyroid problems. The symptoms, like fatigue, are often blamed on pregnancy and postpartum. I actually was diagnosed with postpartum depression but insisted they screen my blood for thyroid issues. They did so

ELSEWHERE ON THE WEB

▶ The Center for Disease Control and Prevention has a really nice frequently-asked-questions (FAQ) section on their page written for the layperson. Check out www .cdc.gov/groupBstrep/gbs/ gen_public_faq.htm. It spells out many of the protocols used for testing mothers, treating those who are positive, and what happens if your baby has group B strep.

only to appease me but were very surprised to find out that I needed thyroid medications and not antidepressants.

Incompetent cervix can cause premature birth. This is where the cervix, or mouth of the uterus is weak and opens prematurely. The cervix can be weak because of prior surgery on the cervix, special medical conditions, like DES exposure, or because of a multiple pregnancy.

Incompetent cervix is a major contributor to second trimester loss. If your cervix opens prematurely, your baby can be born early. If your baby is born early, he is more likely to have complications from the premature birth, including death or life-long disability.

If you have a known risk, like a multiple pregnancy, history of incompetent cervix, or risk factors like DES exposure, your cervix will be monitored via ultrasound for early dilation. If it is found that your cervix is starting to dilate, you will either be placed on bed rest or have a cerclage placed in your cervix.

If you need to have a cerclage put in, you will likely be on bed rest until the cerclage comes out. This is usually done around week thirty-six for most women. You may or may not have your baby immediately. Once treated for incompetent cervix, you will most likely be treated in subsequent pregnancies.

Placenta previa is a problem with your placenta. This is where your placenta is covering all or a part of your cervix. This can cause bleeding in your pregnancy, and if it has not resolved by the time of birth a cesarean section may be the safest way for you to give birth to your baby. Placenta previa is graded in three ways: marginal, partial, or complete.

I get a lot of e-mail from readers right after their week 20 ultrasounds asking about placenta previa. Typically this is when a placenta previa is diagnosed. The good news is that if you are told you have a low-lying placenta at this stage of pregnancy, you have a more than 90-percent chance that the cervix will not be covered at the end of your pregnancy. This means you will be able to have a vaginal birth.

About one in 200 pregnancies is affected by a true placenta previa. They are more common in women who are older, who have had more children, or have had a cesarean section or other type of surgery.

Pregnancy-induced hypertension (PIH) is a problem with blood pressure. PIH affects 5 to 8 percent of all first-time mothers. It has long been one of the biggest problems facing pregnant women.

You may have PIH in any of the following manners:

- High blood pressure only
- High blood pressure with protein in the urine and/or swelling
- High blood pressure with protein in the urine and/or swelling as well as seizures

Your midwife or doctor will screen you for signs of PIH at every prenatal visit. This is one of the reasons why routine prenatal care is very important. Your practitioner will check both your blood pressure and your urine as well as ask you questions about your symptoms. The following symptoms should be reported to your midwife or doctor:

- Rapid weight gain (4–5 lbs in a single week)
- Sudden swelling
- Swelling of your ankles or feet that does not go away after twelve hours of rest

ELSEWHERE ON THE WEB

▶ Mary Shomon is a mom and thyroid expert who also guides the About.com Thyroid site (at http://thyroid.about.com). The site can offer you answers to your questions about thyroid disease during pregnancy. Her common-sense approach to pregnancy and patient advocacy can help you have a safe and healthy pregnancy with thyroid disorders.

- Severe headaches
- Blurry vision or seeing spots in your eyes
- Severe pain over your stomach, under your ribs
- Decrease in the amount of urine

If you do have PIH, your symptoms will be monitored. The goal of your medical team will be to maintain your pregnancy safely as long as possible to allow your baby the most time to grow. Sometimes having PIH will affect how well your baby is growing. If your symptoms become very dangerous and medications like magnesium sulfate and others are not helping control them, or your baby is not growing well enough, your labor may have to be induced or artificially started to best serve you and your baby.

Gestational diabetes starts in pregnancy. Diabetes is where your pancreas does not produce enough insulin or the insulin you do make is not effective in its work. Insulin helps turn blood sugar into energy or fat. Gestational diabetes occurs in about 3 to 5 percent of all pregnant women.

Risk factors for gestational diabetes include the following:

- You are over thirty years old.
- You have a personal or family history of diabetes.
- Your previous baby weighed more than 9 pounds.
- You had a previous stillborn baby.

Usually a screening for gestational diabetes is done around the twenty-eighth week of pregnancy. Your practitioner may decide to do this sooner if you have symptoms or are at high risk for developing gestational diabetes. Gestational diabetes can usually be controlled through diet and exercise. Be sure to ask about a nutrition class if you are diagnosed with gestational diabetes. This will be helpful in maintaining your new lifestyle and managing the disease.

If left unchecked, gestational diabetes can cause you and your baby problems. Your blood sugar can run wild, causing you to experience symptoms like extreme thirst, hunger, or fatigue. However, your baby is at greater risk. If gestational diabetes is left untreated, your excess blood sugar can cause your baby to grow too large. This also results in the risk of birth injury, stillbirth, jaundice, and low blood sugar after birth.

Once you have given birth, gestational diabetes resolves itself, but you are more likely to develop full-blown diabetes later in life. Be sure to talk to your regular family practitioner or internist about your health after pregnancy.

Preterm labor can happen to anyone. Preterm labor can lead to premature birth. About 12 percent of all births in the United States are premature, meaning before week 37 of pregnancy. This is a leading cause of infant mortality. The risk is greatest if you have had a previous baby born prematurely, you are pregnant with multiples, or you have a uterine or cervical anomaly.

Knowing the signs and symptoms of preterm labor drastically improves your chances of getting early treatment. The earlier you are treated for preterm labor, the more likely your practitioner will be able to delay the birth.

The signs you should report immediately include these:

- Contractions that occur ten minutes or less apart (prior to thirty-seven weeks)
- Fluid or blood leaking from the vagina
- Pressure in your pelvis
- Dull backache (may or may not feel rhythmic)

WHAT'S HOT

▶ According to some research, you can also do the gestational diabetes screening with something much more delicious than the typical sugary drinks provided— jelly beans! Using jelly beans in this study actually provided the medical team with very similar reactions to the glucose drinks. The best thing? Women tolerated the jelly beans better.

○ Period-like cramping

○ Abdominal cramping (with or without loose bowels)

If you have any of the above symptoms, you should call your midwife or doctor right away. You will probably be told to rest for an hour on your side and drink two glasses of water and then report back. If symptoms persist, your practitioner will see you, either in the hospital or her office.

You will most likely have a vaginal exam to assess if your cervix is changing. Depending on your symptoms and your cervix, you may be treated with intravenous (IV) hydration therapy and/or medications, given via a shot, an IV, or orally. What medication you need depends on your symptoms, your length of gestation, and other factors. You may require medication for the duration of your pregnancy.

Problems with Baby

Healthy babies are the images most of us see when we imagine our children. No one really expects to have a baby with a problem. But a number of issues can threaten your baby during pregnancy, not to mention birth defects. The good news is that with advances in modern medicine, there is a happy ending for the vast majority of babies with problems.

Amniotic fluid levels matter. There are two conditions that affect pregnant women and their amniotic fluid: oligohydramnios (too little fluid) and polyhydramnios (too much fluid). Both are detected by ultrasound, perhaps after an anomalous uterine measurement. Your midwife or doctor may also detect these conditions by palpating your abdomen.

Amniotic fluid protects your baby in the uterus and allows the baby to move and develop muscles and bones. Your baby also swallows the amniotic fluid and practices breathing with it.

Amniotic fluid comes from a variety of sources. Until week twelve, amniotic fluid is mostly made up of water from you; after that, the fluid is mostly urine from your baby.

Oligohydramnios is a disorder of too little amniotic fluid that affects about 8 percent of mothers. This can be a stand-alone issue, meaning we are not sure what causes it, or it can be caused by something as simple as maternal dehydration or something as complex as kidney problems in your baby.

The problems with having too little amniotic fluid are potentially numerous, though most babies are born healthy with no problems. One of the biggest problems is that your baby has tighter quarters in which to live and move. This can cause growth restriction and even injury to your baby. During labor, too little amniotic fluid can also cause the umbilical cord to get trapped between the baby and the uterus, restricting blood flow to the baby.

While we can't really add water to your uterus during pregnancy, studies do show that in the third trimester, the amount of amniotic fluid is directly linked to maternal hydration. (Though it is interesting to note that at the very end of your pregnancy, a slight decrease in the amount of fluid can be a sign of impending labor.) So be sure to take the amount of water you drink very seriously.

During labor, oligohydramnios may be treated with amnioinfusion. Once your bag of waters has ruptured or is broken by your practitioner, a small catheter can be placed inside the uterus. Then a saline solution is added to surround the baby with more fluid. This can sometimes prevent some of the complications associated with low fluid levels in labor.

Polyhydramnios, a disorder of too much amniotic fluid, affects about 2 percent of pregnant women. You may be sent for an ultrasound because you are measuring large for your gestational age or because your practitioner feels more fluid than baby. Polyhydramnios is more common among mothers with diabetes or who are carrying twins or other higher order multiples. It can also coexist with a congenital malformation of the baby.

During pregnancy, you may not experience any problems from the excess water. Some mothers tell me that they had difficulty breathing and had reflux because of the added pressure in their abdomen on their organs. Be sure to talk to your practitioner about how to treat your symptoms.

Medications that treat maternal disorders like diabetes and some fetal disorders can help reduce excess amniotic fluid. Treatment for polyhydramnios can also be done by selective reduction of the amount of fluid via amniocentesis, but it is more common to just watch and wait. During the labor process, the extra fluid might create more room for the baby to float, meaning it is more likely for the baby to be in a breech position. It can also make a cord prolapse more likely.

Both types of amniotic fluid disorders usually require more testing. This may consist of a series of ultrasounds to assess the amount of fluid around your baby. You might also undergo blood or genetic testing aimed at discovering why you're experiencing difficulties with the amniotic fluid. Your baby will also be more closely monitored, usually via the ultrasounds but also potentially with stress tests and fetal kick counts.

The good news for moms with oligohydramnios or polyhydramnios is that the majority of babies are born with no complications or problems. These are just signs that additional screening is needed. A watchful eye in labor is also suggested, though intervention is not always appropriate. Talk to your practitioner about when intervention may be needed and why.

Growth problems with the baby can occur in pregnancy.
Known as fetal growth restriction (or formerly as intrauterine

▶ Every pregnant woman should be given a large water bottle along with her positive pregnancy test. Staying hydrated can help prevent preterm labor, increase low amniotic fluid levels, and generally make you feel better. You should drink at least 64 ounces of water a day. Fill a large water bottle in the morning and carry it with you all day long. If you do not like plain water, consider adding a bit of lime or lemon to flavor it.

growth retardation [IUGR]), this simply means that for some reason your baby is not growing as it should.

Fetal growth restriction is suspected when your uterus does not grow appropriately, as evidenced by physical examination by your midwife or doctor. You will have ultrasound studies done to confirm the diagnosis and to look for potential reasons for this problem.

Restricted growth can result from maternal complications, such as pregnancy-induced hypertension, pregnancy with multiples, and even inadequate nutrition. Sometimes no cause is found. Treating growth restriction can be as simple as nutritional counseling to increase caloric intake as well as protein. If a problem is found, it will be addressed medically in order for the growth to catch up. If the restriction cannot be reversed, it may be decided that your baby is better off being born now than waiting for labor to begin on its own.

ELSEWHERE ON THE WEB

▶ The March of Dimes is a great source of information on birth defects, with specific and current fact sheets about conditions including Down syndrome, heart defects, spina bifida, and cleft lip and/ or palate. Visit them on the Web at www.marchofdimes .com.

Congenital anomalies are fairly common. About one in twenty-eight women gives birth to a baby with some form of congenital anomaly. This can be a structural defect, or something that affects your baby's functioning, or a metabolic disorder.

Some birth defects, like inherited disorders and gene mutations, have genetic causes. There are also environmental causes, like chemicals you may have been exposed to at certain points in your pregnancy. But more than 60 percent of all genetic defects have unknown causes. Most of the time there is nothing you could have done to prevent the anomaly from occurring.

Bed Rest

The thought behind bed rest is to take the pressure physically or mentally off the mother. This in theory will help her deal with a variety of complications, most frequently issues with preterm labor or high blood pressure. There are a couple of different kinds of bed rest that can be prescribed:

- Modified bed rest
- Strict bed rest
- Complete or hospital bed rest

Modified bed rest is the least restrictive. Usually, modified bed rest means that you should stay home and mostly rest. You may not be able to lift anything heavier than ten pounds. You will not be allowed to do strenuous exercise or walk great distances.

With this type of bed rest, you are usually allowed to leave the house. This might be limited to appointments with your medical team, childbirth classes, and other agreed-upon meetings. Be sure you get the specifics clarified by your doctor or midwife.

Bed rest can be amazingly dull. While the idea of sleeping in every day may once have sounded like a dream come true, bed gets old fast when you're stuck there. Bed rest is not fun for anyone.

Take strict bed rest seriously. It means exactly what it says, to stay in bed. Okay, so you can probably move to the couch during the day, but the premise is the same—you do not move around a whole lot.

This means you get to catch up on your e-mail, your reading list, and a ton of television. Bed rest probably also means that you spend a lot of time fluffing pillows and flipping over from hip to hip. Be sure to schedule visits from friends and family so you can feel like you have something going on.

Set up a station to allow you to stay connected without moving around. Have a collection of books, magazines, the remote control, and the phone brought to your area before your husband leaves for the day. This way you can do most everything from your command center. If you have a laptop, this can also be set up so you can stay connected during the day.

You need to have something to eat as well. Keep light snacks nearby. Think protein, like nuts and peanut butter. You can also do crackers, dried fruit, fresh fruit, and other good food that doesn't need refrigeration. One dad wrote me to say he purchased a small refrigerator to keep upstairs for when he was gone during the day, so his wife didn't have to trek downstairs for lunch.

Complete bed rest is very serious. This is usually done in the hospital because of the specialized treatments that may be needed. Here they can do fetal monitoring as needed as well as other medical treatments. You may need to be placed in the Trendelenberg position, with your feet above your head.

Being in the hospital is no fun. Any visiting-hour restrictions may be relaxed for your spouse so that he can come and go at any time.

Your food will be taken care of, and you might even have some choice in the matter. Be sure to ask for specialty care, like music therapy or healing touch. These can be nice complementary options to the medical management you are already receiving.

Be sure you know the rules of your confinement. No matter what type of bed rest you are on, it is important to understand what is required of you and why. Here are some questions to ask:

- Why am I on bed rest?
- How long am I on bed rest?
- What symptoms do I need to report and to whom?

▶ If you are on bed rest but are allowed to go out occasionally, consider using a wheelchair. You might think I am mad, but after a while stuck in bed, even a trip to the grocery store can be tempting. Most stores have wheelchairs you can borrow. If you are up for a fun baby adventure, consider letting your husband push you around the baby store so you can experience the joys of shopping for baby together.

- Am I allowed up to go to the bathroom?
- Can I negotiate the stairs? How many times a day?
- Are there special exercises I can do?

Relationships get strained when complications occur. It is hard not to feel the stress and strain of pregnancy complications in your relationships. You probably feel helpless and unable to change anything.

Your husband might be the best help, but he might still feel stressed. Now he's Super Mom as well as Super Dad. He's got his own work, the housework, and potentially taking care of the kids added to his plate. Even though he knows that you need to rest and take it easy, his increased load isn't any lighter.

This may all be complicated by the fact he can't really talk about his feelings to his best supporter—you. Not wanting to burden you, he may turn it inward and be more quiet than usual. Try not to take it personally. Offer to listen as objectively as you can and go from there. If this persists or if he is not comfortable talking to you, try to encourage him to seek the confidence of another friend or even a professional if need be.

If you have other kids, they may also feel the strain of complications. The younger they are, the less likely they are to understand why mommy can't play on the floor or chase them around like she used to do. Arrange play dates that get them out of the house or running around. Then save the quiet times for you!

Getting Support When Complications Arise

Most of the time complications are unexpected, often leaving you reeling and trying to figure out what to do and where to go. The best advice I have for you to is to seek support. This support can come in many fashions.

If you have been given a diagnosis that you do not know much about, perhaps you could seek out others with the same issue. You may find that there is a local support group set up to help you. They may offer phone support or information, both of which can be incredibly helpful.

Sometimes you need to talk to a professional. This might be the best way for you to talk about your feelings. Every complication has unique effects on your family. These can change the dynamics of your life as well as how you feel about your life, your family, your baby, and your beliefs.

Such earth-shattering questions and feelings can make you feel out of sorts and depressed. Being able to discuss the situation with a neutral party can be helpful. There may even be someone in your area who specializes in dealing with pregnant women with complications. You can also ask others who have been in the same situation or you can call your local mental health referral agency.

Physical support is important too. You might not be able to care for your home, your kids, or even yourself. This is when you need to enlist the help of others to help run your daily life. Though asking for this help can be difficult, you might have friends or family available to help you with tasks like cooking and cleaning or even child care.

Be sure to accept help when it is offered. People want to help or they would not have offered. If it makes things easier, list all the things you need help doing. When someone offers you support, simply show them the list and let them pick.

ELSEWHERE ON THE WEB

▶ Sidelines (on the Web at www.sidelines.org) is an organization dedicated to helping families through complicated pregnancies. You'll find information on surviving emotionally and mentally as well as handy ways to get your family help while you're down for the count. You can even see if there is a local chapter and potentially get set up with a mentor.

Get Linked

Every day there are strides made toward correcting and preventing certain complications in pregnancy. The Web is a wonderful resource for that information. Here are some links to help you find out more about testing and treatment of pregnancy complications.

PREGNANCY COMPLICATIONS

This section of my site offers you a comprehensive listing of many of the common and not-so-common complications that can occur in pregnancy.

 http://about.com/pregnancy/complications

BIRTH STORIES WITH COMPLICATIONS

Sometimes it's just nice to read about others who have been in a similar situation and to see how everything played out for them. Readers who experienced complications during pregnancy or their birth submitted these stories. Consider submitting yours!

 http://about.com/pregnancy/compbirthstory

Chapter 9

Pregnancy Loss

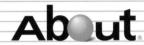

Signs of Trouble

Pregnancy is supposed to be a time of great joy and expectation. The majority of pregnancies will, thankfully, be blissfully trouble-free. However, there will also be pregnancies that experience problems or problematic symptoms. In those cases, you might be left wondering what the heck is going on.

I get a lot of e-mail from women who are worried or frightened by unexpected signs. Some signs or symptoms can be worrisome or downright scary. The good news is that not every nasty or painful symptom should be a cause for alarm. But there are times when you need to know that things are not right.

Here are some of the signs for which that you need to call your doctor or midwife:

- Spotting
- Bleeding

- Dull or sharp aches in the abdomen
- Dull or sharp pain in the back

We all know someone who had signs of trouble in pregnancy but wound up having a wonderful, healthy baby. So it is important, but hard, to remember that not every sign of something wrong means a definite end to the pregnancy. I know how hard this is to remember and believe when you are going through this worrisome period.

A complete disappearance is a potential sign that something is wrong with your pregnancy. This might mean that your annoying morning sickness is suddenly gone, at an inappropriate time. If your breasts were tender, you may notice that it no longer bothers you to wear a bra. It can drive you crazy trying to decide if you're having a good day or if there is something wrong with your pregnancy.

Try to think about it in terms of a collection of symptoms. Do you still have other symptoms? Is it just a qualitative difference? For example, is your morning sickness gone because you've found a way to make it better, while you are still urinating more frequently and having other pregnancy symptoms? Rather than a problem with the pregnancy, this would be an effective way to deal with it.

Try to take all of your symptoms in stride. Remember that different people experience pregnancy in different ways. If you are having problems, it does not necessarily mean anything is terribly wrong. Be sure to report any concerns or questions to your doctor or midwife.

Miscarriage

The miscarriage rate is about 20 percent. This is much higher than anyone would want it to be. And in many cases, the one-in-five number is higher than you would expect. This means that you know someone who has experienced a miscarriage, including me.

Miscarriages are most likely to happen in the first trimester of pregnancy. Though the technical definition includes pregnancy loss up to 20 weeks of gestation, they usually occur before 12 weeks of gestation.

A blighted ovum is also considered a miscarriage. This is where the pregnancy develops as a gestational sac with no baby forming inside the sac. The causes of blighted ovum are the same as with any other miscarriage.

Miscarriage can occur when there are genetic or chromosomal issues with your baby that are incompatible with life. Here are some of the other things that may cause miscarriage:

- Hormonal issues
- Uncontrolled diabetes
- Lupus
- Thyroid disease
- Certain maternal infections, including cytomegalovirus, HIV, or rubella
- Certain illegal drug use
- Alcohol use
- Cigarette smoking
- Exposure to certain toxins

BEFORE YOUR APPOINTMENT

▶ If you have had a previous miscarriage or pregnancy loss, you may be even more concerned before your appointment. This is completely normal. If you need to call your practitioner prior to your appointment, remember that is what she is there for! Don't hesitate to call. She may be able to help ease your concerns.

I want to point out that most of the reasons for miscarriage are beyond the control of you or your practitioner. Suffering a miscarriage does not mean that you will always have problems with pregnancy. Only 1 to 2 percent of couples experience more than one miscarriage.

A lot of my e-mail comes from women asking if they have brought this on themselves. The answer is that it is highly unlikely you've done anything to cause a miscarriage. Miscarriage is not caused by normal everyday life. A fall is unlikely to cause a miscarriage. Using your computer is unlikely to cause a problem with your pregnancy. When in doubt, talk to your practitioner.

Your midwife or doctor will likely ask you questions to help determine what is going on. It is best if you are as specific as possible. Their questions may include information about your last period, your previous pregnancies, and your health in general. Your practitioner may also want to know what you have been doing recently. This might include health, sexual activity, or even recent illnesses.

Testing can be done. A couple of things are standard early in pregnancy when trouble presents itself. You may have repeated blood work done. Your practitioner is looking at hormone levels and how they are changing as well as potentially checking for infection.

Depending on how far along you are, you may also have an ultrasound examination. This will usually be done intravaginally, in which a probe is used to scan the uterus from inside the vagina.

You may also have a physical exam. This is much like your annual gynecologic checkup. Your practitioner will try to figure out how large your uterus is and if your cervix is open. He may also be able to feel other organs, like your ovaries.

Here's what he may be able to tell with all of these tests:

- If your uterus is the appropriate size for your gestational age
- If you have complications with your placenta or its location
- If you have cysts on your ovaries
- If your hCG is rising at an appropriate level
- If you have enough progesterone

The hardest part of all of the testing is the waiting. I hate the waiting. You don't know whether to be happy or to be sad. You don't know what the signs mean that your body is showing. And simply having to have all the tests can be worrisome, even if the results are looking good.

The test results will tell you and your practitioner what the next step should be. Unfortunately, many of the tests have to be repeated to really provide you with any answers. Sometimes the problems you are experiencing are just a normal part of early pregnancy. When you aren't in any immediate danger, waiting keeps you from making a mistake and projecting the worst-case scenario onto your pregnancy when it's just too early to tell anything definitive.

Treatment for Miscarriage   If it is determined that you are indeed miscarrying, there are some different options on how to proceed. The most common option is to let your body take care of itself. The bleeding and pain are then signs of the impending loss. These usually continue for several hours or even a day, until the cervix has opened and the uterus has expelled the tissue.

This can be frightening, particularly if you do not know what to expect. Be sure to ask your doctor or midwife how much bleeding is normal. They may ask you to save any tissue that comes out. They may also prescribe you pain relief.

This expectant management is used the majority of the time in miscarriage. But there are reasons, such as excessive bleeding or tissue left in the uterus, that you might be asked about undergoing surgical management.

Surgical management is usually done in the form of a dilation and curettage (D&C). This is a fairly simple and straightforward surgery. The cervix, if not already opened in the process of miscarriage, will be dilated. Then the doctor cleans out the inside of the uterus. This is normally a very quick procedure. Many are done in the hospital as day surgery, with general anesthesia or sedation.

You will usually stay wherever you had your surgery for about an hour or two. The nurses will check your vital signs and assess your bleeding. You may still spot, but your bleeding should be diminished in most cases. Be sure to ask how much bleeding is too much.

TOOLS YOU NEED

▶ Reading about the experiences of others or finding a ritual for yourself can be very comforting. The books I most commonly recommend are *A Silent Sorrow,* by Perry Lynn Moffit; *Miscarriage: Women Sharing from the Heart,* by Marie Allen and Shelly Marks; and *Empty Cradle, Broken Heart: Surviving the Death of Your Baby,* by Deborah L. Davis.

You may experience some discomfort or cramping. You may be prescribed pain medication or given an over-the-counter remedy. The most common side effects are usually from the anesthesia. These can include drowsiness, nausea, vomiting, and a disoriented feeling. Remember to keep another adult with you for the first few hours after surgery.

Miscarriage Recovery   The physical recovery from miscarriage is usually considered uncomfortable. Some of your discomfort comes from mental and emotional pain as well.

You will probably experience cramping for a day or two after the physical completion of the miscarriage. I found this to be much like severe menstrual cramps that gradually got easier to deal with as time went on. You can also treat it with over-the-counter medications that you might usually use for menstrual cramps, like ibuprofen.

You will probably continue to bleed for a week or two after your miscarriage. This is the lining of the uterus leaving your body in the process of healing. The bleeding should get lighter and become spotting. The further along you were in your pregnancy, the longer you are likely to bleed. During this time period you should use only menstrual pads and not tampons. Using tampons could lead to an infection of the uterus.

The next time you bleed should be your normal menstrual cycle. This will usually happen between three and eight weeks after your miscarriage. After this cycle, you can begin to use tampons again.

Infection is the most common complication after a miscarriage. To avoid infection you should refrain from putting anything into your vagina. This includes tampons and douching. If you are bleeding heavily, it is usually advised that you shower rather than take a tub bath. You should also avoid sex until after you have stopped bleeding.

ELSEWHERE ON THE WEB

▶ SHARE (on the Web at www.nationalshareoffice .com) is an organization designed to help you emotionally deal with the end of your pregnancy, no matter at what point it ended. There is a free newsletter with informative articles for all members of the family as well as a memorial section. SHARE also sponsors Memorial Walks to Remember and educational offerings to help the public learn more about the pain that comes from the death of your baby and how best to help.

The physical recovery will progress from the low point to feeling better each day. You may feel weak afterward, possibly due to blood loss. If you are worried, be sure to ask your doctor or midwife to screen you for anemia. Most practitioners will want to see you back in their office for a follow-up exam about six weeks after your miscarriage.

Testing can be done after miscarriage.   This testing is usually not recommended until after you've had at least two or three early losses or one or two second- or third-trimester losses. Talk to your practitioner about whether testing is right for you or not.

Testing may consist of blood work for you and your partner to test for genetic disease or even infection. It might be a vaginal exam and ultrasound to see the condition of your uterus and ovaries.

Ectopic Pregnancy

A pregnancy that is located anywhere other than the uterus is known as an ectopic pregnancy. You may have also heard it called a tubal pregnancy because many of these pregnancies grow in the fallopian tubes.

Ectopic pregnancies are the leading cause of death in the mother in the first trimester, as the pregnancy is developing in a place that is dangerously small to house it for any length of time. If this pregnancy ruptures, you will bleed internally and need emergency medical attention.

There are some common risk factors for ectopic pregnancy. Hopefully if you have any of the following risk factors, you have been briefed on your increased chances of ectopic pregnancy:

- Pelvic inflammatory disease (PID)
- Tubal ligation (had your tubes tied)
- Intrauterine device (IUD) in place

ASK YOUR GUIDE

Can the baby also be tested after a miscarriage?

▶ Testing the baby for abnormalities is done sometimes. This is usually the case if you have had multiple miscarriages. Some women find it difficult to save any tissue that comes out to bring to their doctor or midwife. If you choose to do this, simply use a clean container that you don't need back, like a small plastic bowl with a lid.

- Previous abdominal/pelvic surgery (including cesarean section)
- Infertility
- Endometriosis
- Previous ectopic pregnancy

If this pregnancy grows beyond the size of the space, it can rupture and cause massive internal bleeding. This is why being able to diagnose and treat an ectopic pregnancy is so important to your health and future fertility.

Ectopic pregnancies can grow in a couple of places: your cervix, your ovary, your abdomen, and your fallopian tube. Each of these places poses a problem for your pregnancy.

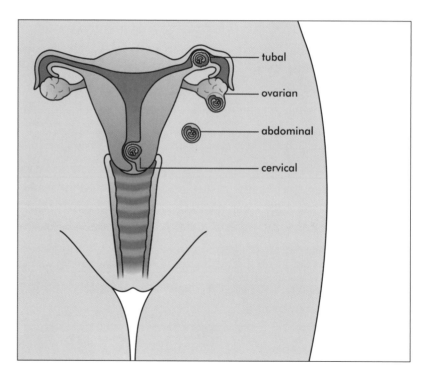

▲ Types of ectopic pregnancy

Signs of an ectopic pregnancy include these:

- Vaginal bleeding
- Abdominal pain
- Shoulder pain
- Weakness
- Dizziness

Sometimes ectopic pregnancies can be detected by blood tests, though these are not as accurate as we would hope. This usually happens very early on as you see an abnormal rise in the hCG levels. Ultrasound can also be used to detect an ectopic pregnancy, but only after about five to six weeks gestation. Occasionally surgery has to be done to see if there is any distention in the fallopian tubes or other areas to find the source of the symptoms.

If an ectopic pregnancy is found early enough and you meet other requirements, you may be offered a medication to help resolve the pregnancy. The medication most often used is called methotrexate. This medication is given by injection and causes the pregnancy to be reabsorbed into your body.

If you are not a candidate for methotrexate, or the ectopic pregnancy has already ruptured, you may require surgery. Surgery is done to help stave off bleeding and remove the pregnancy. Unfortunately we have not been able to find a way to remove a pregnancy from one location and relocate it to another location.

This type of surgery is usually done with general anesthesia. General anesthesia is usually given via intravenous medications, though sometimes a gas is used. The good news is that you will be asleep and not feel any of the surgery. Any other medications you may need during the surgery, as well as fluids, can be given through your IV as well.

What other symptoms can be expected after ectopic surgery?

▶ Feelings of weakness or dizziness can be common after ectopic surgery. It may be from the loss of blood making you anemic. Immediately after the surgery, it may be from pain medication or even the anesthesia itself. Take life slowly once you get home from the hospital. Taking some time off from work will enable you to rest and let your body heal from surgery. It will also give you some emotional space to deal with your grief.

In surgery the decision may be made to remove the affected fallopian tube and/or ovary. For many women, the loss of one tube or ovary does not have a huge affect on their fertility. With the removal of the tube, the pregnancy is also removed. Any additional necessary repairs are made during the surgery.

Recovering from surgery is not a pleasant task. Much of your recovery will depend on the type of surgery you had. Most women will have a laparoscopy. This is a smaller set of three incisions, usually called Band-Aid surgery because of the less invasive route. The other type of surgery is called a laparotomy, which involves a larger incision above the pubic hair, much like a cesarean section incision.

Both of these are abdominal surgeries. You will feel sore around your incisions. These may be closed with either sutures or staples, depending on different factors. I found splinting my incision with a small pillow helped me get out of bed sooner. The slight pressure against my skin kept me from feeling like my insides were going to hit the floor if I stood up.

You will usually spend a night in the hospital. While there you will learn to care for your incisions. This includes looking for infection. The incisions may weep fluids, but should not be bright red or warm to the touch, nor should you run a fever. If you have any of these symptoms, call your practitioner immediately.

After taking time off from work and some physical and emotional rest, you can slowly add your daily routines back into your life, starting with the smallest of tasks and working your way up. If you have staples, these may be removed about ten to fourteen days after surgery. After this checkup, your doctor or midwife will talk to you about physical abilities and exercise.

Most of the women I talk to say that it took about six to eight weeks before they physically felt like themselves again. Remember to take it slowly and not to expect too much from your body physically or emotionally.

If you also lost your tube during surgery, you may have additional feelings of loss. I've talked to women who said they felt "lopsided" on the side their tube and/or ovary was missing from. They knew that the few ounces of a body part didn't really make that much physical difference, but the mental issues were causing these feelings.

Late Pregnancy Loss

Late pregnancy loss is usually defined as after twenty weeks of gestation. This is also known as stillbirth. Stillbirth is where your baby dies before being born. It is even possible to have it happen in labor.

About one in 200 pregnancies ends in stillbirth, and about a third of all stillbirths are from unknown causes. There are numerous potential causes of stillbirth, including these:

- Placental problems
- Growth problems
- Infection
- Severe trauma
- Maternal complications, such as high blood pressure or diabetes

Stillbirth is diagnosed by ultrasound to determine if your baby's heart is still beating. This may be a routine ultrasound, or you may be going in because of a specific problem. Many times, mothers report a decrease in fetal movement and the doctor or midwife listens for the heartbeat. If it can't be heard, an ultrasound is ordered.

If you have been diagnosed with a stillborn baby prior to labor, you will have a couple of choices about your baby's birth. Though in most cases it is normal for labor to begin on its own within about two weeks, many midwives and doctors will let you choose to be

▶ After being diagnosed with a stillborn baby, you will want to take some time to think about the situation. Before you see your doctor or midwife again, you will want to formulate some questions about how you will be cared for during labor. If you were planning a birth center or home birth, will you have to now go to the hospital? Will you need to use or avoid certain medications? Who can you have with your during your labor and birth? What are the hospital policies about caring for your baby after birth? What will you be provided in the way of emotional support?

induced. The point here is that you do not need to make an immediate decision in the majority of cases.

You may need time to comprehend the horrible news you have just been given. You may want time to settle your family at home to prepare for the birth, as with older children. Or you may be waiting for a special relative or friend to come be with you. These are all options for the majority of women.

Stillbirth and Labor   Labor and birth are essentially the same for a woman who is giving birth to a still baby. The contractions will come and your cervix will open. You will have the same support as in any labor, such as the presence of your husband or a doula, massage, breathing or other relaxation techniques, or medication.

No fetal monitor is used during your labor. Some hospitals do request that you occasionally submit to contraction monitoring, especially if medications like Pitocin or pain relief drugs are in use. These are to monitor your health or the strength of your contractions.

You may choose to make different decisions about this labor than if your baby had been alive. For example, if you were previously planning on having an unmedicated birth to avoid exposing your baby to medications, you may not care about this anymore. I have also spoken to several moms who had been planning on epidurals until they found out their babies had died. Each of these moms chose to have no pain medication; they felt like it physically tied them to the experience more.

This decision to use or not use medication in labor is yours. The only thing I would caution you against is the use of medications that leave you with trouble remembering the labor, birth, or the immediate postpartum period. Mothers who have done so complain later that they wish their memories of their baby were clearer.

The pushing phase of labor may take a bit longer. This is because normally your baby would help himself be born by twisting and turning. There is also an emotional barrier many women experience at this point. You may feel like as long as you can hold your baby inside your body he or she is safe, making you hold back intentionally or unintentionally from giving birth. This is a completely normal feeling.

An induction of labor may be medically necessary or your choice. Some women have written to me that while they would have preferred a natural start to labor, that they could not fathom walking around, obviously pregnant, and yet knowing their baby wasn't alive. Talk to your midwife or doctor about the types of induction that are options for you, if this is a choice you wish to make.

Cesareans are not usually done simply because a baby is stillborn. These are surgeries that should be done only in the event that the labor and birth are proving difficult. The added danger of the surgery for the mom is usually not worth the risk. There are also additional risks to future pregnancies after a cesarean, including infertility (subfertility), placenta previa, and an increased risk of stillbirth.

Holding Your Baby   After your baby is born, you will be given time to hold your baby. It is normal to feel very sad and cry. Those around you may also be crying, even your practitioners. You should consider having photos taken of your baby. Many hospitals will do this automatically, but feel free to take your own as well. You might consider having photos of you and your spouse holding the baby.

Dress your baby. Name your baby. Cuddle your baby. Do whatever you need to do to personally cope with the situation. This will be your chance to hold your baby physically. It is normal to

TOOLS YOU NEED

▶ After a stillbirth, be sure to take as many pictures as you can. Buy a camera from the hospital gift shop or even a nearby store if you must. Don't worry about sad expressions or how anyone looks. Be sure to get lots of pictures of your baby up close, including undressed. Remember small parts too, such as hands, feet, and bottom. These will be important to you later. You should also collect anything your baby used while there, like clothes or blankets. Also ask for several footprint cards. You can put these away and look at them later if you choose or just know they are safely in your home.

be worried or frightened. Have a nurse or social worker help you if you need to do so.

There are normally no time limits on how long you will have with your baby. You can usually have as much time as you need. The baby will normally stay at the hospital as long as you do.

Many hospitals will put a small card on the outside of your door to signify your loss. This will prevent well-meaning hospital workers from asking questions or being unintentionally disrespectful. You may also have the option of a shorter stay in the hospital or staying in a part of the hospital that is not a postpartum floor.

You will be asked many questions during the first few hours after your baby is stillborn. You may be asked about funeral arrangements or services. Feel free to ask for help. The hospital will probably have a social worker help you. But do not hesitate to ask for your clergy to come to assist you.

You may decide to delay the services until after you are out of the hospital. You might decide to hold no services or hold a small service in the hospital. There is not a single right answer for everyone.

Physical Recovery Postpartum will physically feel the same as with any other pregnancy. You will still have bleeding, or lochia. Your uterus will need about six weeks to shrink back down into your pelvis. Your breasts will still make milk.

There are a couple of thoughts on postpartum milk production after a stillbirth. You may choose to hurry up and try to dry up your milk supply by binding your breasts or wearing a tight bra. You may also choose to pump for a few days to allow the hormones to help you adjust. You may also decide to pump your breasts and donate your milk. Be sure to ask if this is an option in your area. Some mothers have written to me telling me how wonderful it felt to know that their milk was saving another baby. The choice is totally up to you. A lactation consultant will be able to help you choose the best option for you and help you ease out of milk production with as little pain as possible.

You will follow up with your doctor or midwife at the normal six-week postpartum visit, unless you require one earlier. At this visit, your practitioner will check your body to ensure you are healing physically. She may also go over test results with you or review any questions you have about your labor and birth.

Typically a pap smear and breast exam are also done at this visit. You may also discuss birth control. This would be the perfect time to ask questions such as these:

- Will I need any other follow-up physical care?
- How long do you recommend I wait before conceiving again?
- Do you know of any resources or materials for women in my situation?
- How will this affect future pregnancies?
- Will you need to do any testing prior to my conceiving again?

Testing Sometimes the cause of your baby's death may be obvious. Other times it is not obvious at all. Figuring out what happened may take a bit longer than you would hope, sometimes months.

There may be blood tests done on you to check for infections or diseases. You may or may not have the option of an autopsy of your baby. (Religious and medical reasons may play into this decision.) The placenta will be thoroughly examined, including blood cultures. Again, no reason is found for about a third of the cases of stillbirth.

ELSEWHERE ON THE WEB

▸ You or anyone in your family can request free bereavement information from the March of Dimes for the loss of a baby from conception until one month of age. Visit www.march ofdimes.com for more information. These helpful pamphlets talk about the stages of grief and ways to remember your baby. They may also be available from your doctor or midwife.

Trying Again

After having your pregnancy end or your baby die, it is normal to feel skittish about trying again. Part of you may desire to become pregnant immediately, while another part may never want to experience pregnancy again. These are both normal feelings.

You should talk to your doctor or midwife about how long you should wait before getting pregnant again. Part of this will depend on factors like the following:

- How far along you were in pregnancy
- The reason for your loss (if known)
- Whether you required medical intervention
- Your physical health
- Your fertility status

You may be asked to wait longer if you gave birth, particularly if you had to have a cesarean section. This is because your body does not know the difference between a live birth and a stillbirth in terms of how it recovers. We know from medical studies that your body is healthiest with about eighteen months between pregnancies. This waiting time may be more critical for some than for others.

A New Pregnancy   A new pregnancy will bring about many emotions. You may feel frightened. You might feel elated. You will probably feel both. Probably the most important thing to remember is that each pregnancy is completely new and different.

Emotionally, a new pregnancy will be difficult. There will be many points at which you may worry about your pregnancy. Some may be directly tied to your original loss. Other points of worry may be new, as you have now lost the innocence you had before your loss.

I can remember telling one of my doctors that I simply wished I could sleep for the first trimester and wake up in the second

▶ I highly recommend the book *Trying Again: A Guide to Pregnancy After Miscarriage, Stillbirth or Infant Loss.* I took part in some of the discussions surrounding the development of this book, which is for women who have had miscarriages but want to try again to have a baby. The women who contributed had wonderful insights and really knew what it felt like to be there. I gained so much from these women. The best part is that this book was put together with the loving hand of Ann Douglas, who has experienced pregnancy loss herself.

trimester. I was merely voicing the fact that the first trimester was scary and I would do anything to avoid it. It is perfectly all right to have these types of feelings. The key is to find someone to help you through them. This can be your spouse, a friend, a support group, your practitioner, or even better, all of the above.

Simply surviving the next pregnancy is the key. Dealing with the worries and emotions that creep up daily is difficult. There will be days you are very sad. This is normal and not a reflection of how you will be forever.

You may feel like you are having trouble bonding with this baby prenatally. This may be because you are afraid of another loss or because you have failed to even really accept that you are pregnant. I had this experience in one of my pregnancies. We had had several losses in a row, and I just couldn't fathom that we'd ever have a baby. My husband actually felt the same thing!

We went through all the motions of having a baby. Finally, around the eighth month of pregnancy, it hit us. I remember crying and crying. I felt horribly guilty for having cheated our baby out of nearly an entire pregnancy. Needless to say we worked very hard on bonding during the last six weeks of my pregnancy by talking and writing letters to the baby.

Here are the keys to surviving a new pregnancy:

- Find support from others who have been there.
- Don't stress about being stressed.
- Try to enjoy your pregnancy, even if just a little bit.
- Remember every pregnancy is different.
- Go ahead and plan—it's okay.
- Love and accept your new baby.

Planning your next labor and birth can be emotionally taxing. It may become hard to separate out the fact from the emotion.

▶ Talk to your midwife or doctor about how a future pregnancy will be different. Will there be other tests performed? Extra monitoring? What will you need to know about a new pregnancy? They should give you answers that allay your fears. If not, you need to sit down and talk some more. A new pregnancy will stress you and strain you; you don't need to add the worry that your practitioner doesn't support you to the mix.

Try to find a neutral party to discuss your options with you. This is usually not a member of your family or your medical team. You might consider a doula or childbirth educator to help you formulate questions to ask of your medical team to help you make decisions that are not based on fear.

If you labored before, you may worry about having negative emotions come up in labor. The same is true if you have had a previous cesarean birth. Simply going through the same steps can bring back old memories. And it can be difficult to know that you are not in the same situation as before.

The moms who write me say that hearing their baby cry was high on their list of things that made it real for them. Be sure to share what you are looking forward to with your doctor or midwife. Hopefully they will ask, so they can help ensure a positive memory for you, but offer it up for them if they don't.

Consider planning something special for the birth or right after to celebrate the new life while remembering the lives that were lost before. This can be something very simple. It can be a birth announcement that includes the names of any previous children on it. It might be a special ceremony you design that others participate in. My husband and I simply chose to have a few moments absolutely alone with our new baby as soon as possible after birth. We cried and were sad for what we had previously lost and yet were thrilled and overwhelmed with the new life in our arms.

Your support system will help you through the normal issues of postpartum. Late-night feedings, sleep deprivation, and the hormonal roller coaster we call postpartum are all a part of the game. Don't hesitate to talk to your doctor, midwife, doula, pediatrician, grief counselor, friends, or family for help in dealing with a new baby or the memories of your loss.

Get Linked

DON'T SAY THAT!

This article is really for everyone else in your life. I encourage you to print it out or send the URL to your friends and loved ones. It's a nice primer on what not to say to someone whose baby just died. It can be a great starting point for those hard-to-have discussions or simply a way to let them know what you don't need right now. Feel free to add your own.

 http://about.com/pregnancy/dontsaythat

PREGNANCY LOSS

The information here spans a wide variety of topics dealing with different types of pregnancy loss. From stories of personal loss to resources to help you cope with the physical issues related to miscarriage, there is something here for everyone.

 http://about.com/pregnancy/pregnancyloss

ONE MISCARRIAGE, ONE MAN, ONE WOMAN

Men and women grieve differently. It's a fact. But trying to grieve the same loss simultaneously can be very difficult on your relationship. Here one man and one woman each explore their thoughts about the same loss.

 http://about.com/pregnancy/miscarriage

Chapter 10

Journey to Birth: Preparing for Labor

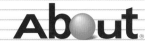

Picking the Right Childbirth Class for You

Okay, so you've probably got a few images in your mind of what childbirth class looks like. It's a bunch of pregnant women lying around like beached whales doing funny breathing. Am I right? This couldn't be further from the actual truth for most childbirth classes.

The whole point behind childbirth class is to prepare you and everyone on your support team for the process of labor and birth, as well as the early days postpartum. Childbirth class is where you can learn while not being pressured by policy, practitioner, or anything else. You can sit with an open mind and hear all sides of the story.

In childbirth class, you can expect to learn about the following topics:

- How to time contractions
- How to tell if you're in labor
- Positioning to make labor and birth more comfortable and easier
- Support for birth from family, doulas, and your birth team
- Informed consent—what it is and how to get it
- Relaxation techniques
- Comfort measures for labor, birth, and postpartum
- Normal labor and birth
- Breastfeeding
- Complications of labor
- Medications (such as Pitocin, epidural, IV medications)
- Operative delivery (cesarean section, forceps, and vacuum)
- Postpartum warning signs
- Normal postpartum physical and emotional changes
- Breastfeeding
- New baby care

While these are the basics of a childbirth class, some classes offer more in-depth information on more topics. For example, some may cover pregnancy nutrition or exercise in addition to other topics. These are all bonuses, but remember you need the extra time to cover these topics. A few hours is not long enough to cover a handful of these subjects. You should choose a class with a minimum of twelve contact hours, though more hours are even better.

The truth is there is not one perfect class for everyone. I like to think of childbirth classes as a core class, like the list above, and additions to that core. These additions might be a class that covers a topic in more detail, like a breastfeeding class or multiple pregnancy, or an additional topic that is handy to have, like infant CPR.

There are many things you need to consider when taking a childbirth class, such as the following:

- When is the class taught?
- Where is the class taught? Hospital, home, office, birth center?
- Is the instructor certified by a recognized childbirth educator organization, like Lamaze, Bradley, or ICEA?
- Is there a limit on the number of couples in class?
- Are multiple techniques used in teaching?
- Does the class include information you need?
- Is there any obvious bias in the class? (Think, "Use our hospital, it's better" type bias.)
- How many students choose to go without medication?

The shortest number of hours doesn't necessarily equal the best instruction. In our hectic lives, many of us wait to find a childbirth class, cramming it into the ninth month or into the fewest possible hours. One thing we know about any kind of instruction is that the more hours you spend face to face with your teacher and other students, the more likely you are to retain the information.

Another important factor is how the classes are scheduled, in as the layout of the hours. A twelve-hour weekend course, for instance, is not going to be the same quality of learning as you would get from a twelve-hour course taught over the course of six weeks. This gives your brain more time to process new material.

Remember, you get what you pay for. There are places where you can take a childbirth class for free. These types of

ASK YOUR GUIDE

I have already taken childbirth classes for a previous baby. Do I really need another class?

▶ Absolutely! You have to remember that each set of classes focuses on this pregnancy. You are likely to hear things a different way now that you have been through labor. It is also a great way to gather your thoughts for how you want this birth to be alike or different from your first birth. My husband and I found taking classes a nice way to really focus on the newest member of our family, something not so easy to do with another child at home. Think of it as date night out with your new baby!

▶ One of the things I hear from many of the students in my classes and from people online is that they really enjoy class visits from recent graduates. This means a couple comes back to talk about their birth and early postpartum experience. They give you an opportunity to ask them questions about nearly anything that you want to hear from someone who has recently been there and done that. Be sure to ask teachers you interview if they offer this as a part of their class.

childbirth classes are usually taught by hospitals, birth centers, or practitioner's offices. While the price might be tempting, ask yourself some questions about the class before you sign up.

Are the classes overly large? An ideal childbirth class should be between four and eight couples, and never more than twelve couples. The more students, the harder it is to learn.

Are the classes taught by certified childbirth instructors? Believe it or not, simply being a nurse in labor and delivery doesn't give you all the information or knowledge you need to lead an effective childbirth class. Even though these nurses may have a lot of knowledge to share, their employer or a lack of knowledge of adult education might limit what they can teach you.

If a childbirth instructor is certified by a national or international body, she has met a set of standards on how to teach adults about all aspects of childbirth and not just the ones that your local facility finds important. A certified childbirth educator also has to continue to learn by maintaining a certain number of hours in refreshing her knowledge and keeping her skills sharp by recertifying with the organization who certified her.

Affiliated classes aren't always neutral. Sometimes the message of each class has a spin placed on it by the hospital or location. For example, some hospitals do not allow their childbirth educators to explain the risks of an epidural, for fear you wouldn't accept these risks. Other places might push certain procedures or features on you, not because they're in your best medical interest but more as a marketing tool. Childbirth class as a marketing tool doesn't always work well. You need to find classes that are neutral and teach you everything there is to know in an unbiased manner.

One thing that I find important is that it not be a fear-based class. What I mean by this is that the childbirth educator is not giving you information in a threatening way, with what I call the healthy baby card. "If you don't have continuous internal fetal monitoring, you won't have a healthy baby. You want a healthy baby, right?" Who is going to say no? But the truth is the monitoring isn't going to ensure a healthy baby. In fact, it may lead to more complications for the normal, low-risk woman. You need all the facts to make your own decision.

Here are some questions to ask your childbirth educator:

- With whom are you certified? What are the certification requirements?
- What is your philosophy of teaching childbirth classes?
- Do you attend births on a regular basis?
- What is your teaching style? Is your class lecture-based or interactive?
- Will you show videos?
- Is there a childbirth class reunion?
- Can I talk to some of your graduates?

In the end, the class you pick will hopefully be a good fit for you and your partner. If you do find your way into a class that is not a good match, be sure to talk to the educator. Give her a chance to right the wrongs. If it is still not working, do not hesitate to find a different class.

Support in Labor

The need for support, for surrounding yourself with people to care for you and help you during your labor and birth, is so important. I cannot stress this enough. You need to have those you love around. You need to have knowledgeable people to care for you and your baby's medical needs, and you need someone to care for your emotional and physical needs.

Obviously your family and friends work well for filling the loving roles. This helps you to stay calm and know that those around you

ASK YOUR GUIDE

When is the best time to take a childbirth class?

▶ I recommend that you be registered for a childbirth class by the time you are twenty weeks pregnant. Ideally you would finish your classes prior to week thirty-four or thirty-five. This means you're not left scrambling at the end of your pregnancy to find the ideal class for you or settling for one you don't really want. And you have time to use the information presented before the baby is born.

are familiar. You can be assured that they are excited about the birth or your baby and care for you.

The medical team you select will be there to care for your medical needs. This would include your medical care in pregnancy and for the labor and birth. This is your midwife or doctor and the medical team at your place of birth. This can include nurses, lab workers, lactation consultants, and others.

The last area that you need to have covered is your physical and emotional needs. For this I would highly recommend a doula. A doula is someone who can focus only on your physical comfort and emotional needs and who is not emotionally involved with becoming a father. Your doctor or midwife will need to focus on your medical care and that of your baby. Your nurses will also be focused on the medical aspects of your care. Your family and friends will focus on you but will also be emotionally thinking of their new roles as the baby's father or aunt, as the case may be. These people are also less likely to have the hands-on knowledge and support that a doula will bring to your labor.

By using a doula, you will drastically reduce the likelihood of many complications, including cesarean section, the use of Pitocin, forceps, episiotomy, and others. Using a doula can also help you have a shorter, more comfortable labor.

How does a doula do all of these amazing things? A doula is trained to help you use your body's instincts by selected positions that help you be more comfortable in labor and to help labor progress more quickly. Her training also includes information on a variety of comfort measures like massage, heat and cold therapy, and others to help you work with your labor.

In complicated labors, while less common in doula-attended births, she can help you by providing you with information that will help you communicate with the hospital or birth center staff and your practitioner.

Find a list of doulas in your area. See if you can get some personal recommendations from mothers who had birth experiences similar to the one you wish to have. You can also look online for lists of doulas in your area. Narrow down that list by conducting phone interviews and then have a couple of face-to-face interviews. Questions you may want to ask a doula include these:

- What is your training?
- Are you certified or working toward certification?
- What are your fees and what does that include? Prenatal visits? Labor? Postpartum?
- Do you have a backup doula available for times when you may not be available?
- What is your philosophy of birth?
- Have you ever worked with my practitioner or at my place of birth?
- May I contact your references?

Certification shows that the doula has met a minimum amount of training and is serious about her work. While having a long history of attending births is a positive thing, as is previous work with your doctor or midwife, be sure to not overlook someone that you and your partner just really connect with during an interview. Sometimes that connection is the best indicator of the right doula for your family.

It's All about Positioning

Position, position, position! It is the key to a more comfortable labor. Being able to assume different positions based on the feedback from your body and your baby will help your labor flow faster and allow you greater comfort during this time. While the positions you choose should come naturally to you, sometimes we resist them or feel like we should do something else that is expected of us.

Your body will give you a really good lead to follow in labor if you will listen. Practicing these positions ahead of time will help strengthen muscles used in birth and prepare you mentally as well. I teach them in childbirth class so that couples can physically practice them together so they don't feel strange once labor starts. It also helps you remember that labor is an active process, not a passive event.

Standing with your partner is a very nice position. Here you get the benefit of gravity from being upright as well as the benefit of holding on to your honey. This can also be done as slow dancing, which works really well in early labor as a way to pass some time or late in labor when you need a bit of support when on your feet. This position gives you the following benefits:

- Close contact with your support people, like your husband
- Upright position for labor progress
- Movement to help ease discomforts

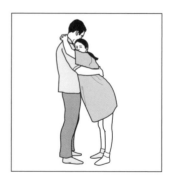

▲ Leaning position

Leaning forward helps tip the baby into your pelvis. This can help alleviate back labor. It also feels great. This can be done standing and leaning onto a person or an object like a birth ball. Or you can do it sitting and leaning forward or even kneeling, with the following benefits:

- Helps encourage baby into your pelvis
- Promotes relaxation
- Can be used in between or during contractions

Hands and knees works well during the later stages of labor. It is a great position for you to assume if you need a break from the contractions. While it doesn't stop them, it does take the edge off. It is also nice because it allows your support people more access to your back for a massage, as well as other benefits:

- Helps rotate a baby to the optimal position
- Can provide pain relief, particularly for back labor
- Is a gravity-neutral position, to slow a fast birth

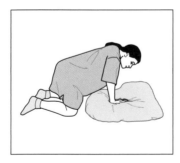

▲ On all fours

ASK YOUR GUIDE

Is there one position for labor that works the best?

▶ Surprisingly, no. There isn't one position that works best for everyone. When you try different positions in labor you will find some provide more comfort than others. These positions are the ones you should use. That said, I suggest that you completely avoid lying on your back. This position is counterproductive and often painful for laboring women. It also impedes the birth process. So get up and get moving!

Once your baby is engaged, you can squat. Squatting takes a bit of practice before labor to get the most benefit. Use a person or a chair to help you learn the position. When you're in labor, you can squat during a contraction and then use a different position in between contractions to help ease the stress on your legs. This position also provides these benefits:

- Opens the pelvis more than other positions
- Uses gravity to help pull the baby down
- Can help protect your perineum from tears
- Works well for pushing

Sitting on a ball is easy. It is also very comfortable. Just like sitting up on any chair, you can use a ball to help ease your body in labor. The benefit of the ball is that it is much more flexible on your bottom and allows more movement in your pelvis. Beside freeing up your back for a massage, it offers these benefits:

- Wide variety of uses in labor and birth
- When used in sitting positions, gravity helps the baby descend
- Encourages movement in mom

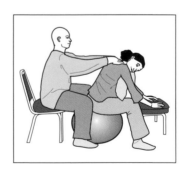

▲ Sitting on a ball

Sitting backwards in a chair feels great! Just throw a pillow over the back of the chair and lean onto it. This position helps you open your legs and stretch as well as being upright or mostly upright. It also offers these benefits:

- Use of gravity helps the labor progress
- Lets you rest your legs
- Gives your supporters access to your back for massage

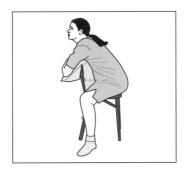

▲ Sitting backwards in a chair

Choose an upright position for pushing and giving birth. No matter what positions you've used in labor, the choice for birth can be different. As in labor, an upright position will help use gravity to ease and speed the birth. Nearly any position that you could have used in labor works well for giving birth. The most commonly used positions for birth are these:

- Squatting
- Hands and knees
- Sitting, leaning forward

TOOLS YOU NEED

▶ A birth ball or physiotherapy ball is a wonderful tool for labor. I used one as a replacement for my desk chair the last few weeks of my pregnancy with the twins, and I felt so much better. It had a forgiving seat to ease the strain on my back and bottom. It also forced me to have good posture, which made my back feel much better. These same reasons make it a blessing for labor. So if you don't have one, go get one now!

Each of these positions helps to use your body to its fullest advantage. This allows the straightest path for your baby to be born. Many women say that these positions also felt better than the reclining alternatives. The good news is that your choice of position can actually help prevent some complications or interventions, including episiotomy and dystocia, the slowing of labor.

Common Interventions in Labor and Birth

Labor and birth are normal processes, but there are times when we intervene. Sometimes these interventions are done to help labor, while at other times they are simply done as a part of a routine. With routine interventions, we often don't think about why they are being done or what chain reaction is set off by interfering with a natural process without good cause.

IV therapy is often used in labor. The purpose is to rehydrate someone who has been dehydrated or to provide access to your veins should medications become necessary quickly. This is done in many hospitals as a matter of routine.

It will be mandatory if you desire medications, are high risk, or are having surgery. Because an IV can limit your mobility, you can ask to have a saline lock placed. This provides access to your veins without any tubing attached to inhibit your movement. If IV therapy is needed for medications that do not run continuously, you can have the medication given and then have the tubing removed again, without being stuck. This is a perfect compromise should you need antibiotics in labor.

In a birth center, IVs are not done on a routine basis, nor are they in the home birth setting; however, most practitioners do have the ability to do this should they need to for some other reason. Be sure to ask your doctor or midwife what circumstance that would be.

Fetal monitoring is something done in all labors. This is to ensure that your baby is doing well. There are several methods of fetal monitoring:

- Auscultation
- External electronic fetal monitoring
- Internal electronic fetal monitoring

With auscultation, the nurse, midwife, or doctor listens to your baby with a Doppler, fetoscope, or other device. This is very much like what happens during your prenatal visits. It can be done while you are in any position and affords the person listening the ability to tell how your baby is reacting to labor. The benefits of using this form of monitoring are that you are not tethered to a machine. You also have a human on the other end deciphering the input rather than a machine.

External fetal monitoring (EFM) uses a pressure transducer to monitor your contractions and an ultrasound device to record your baby's heartbeat. These are strapped onto your abdomen using two belts, with lines back to the machine. This limits your ability to move and change positions while you are being monitored.

Intermittent monitoring with electronic fetal monitoring is possible. You simply need to remove the belts and walk around or assume other positions. A nurse or your practitioner will watch the monitor to determine how your baby is doing, usually from outside the labor room. This type of monitoring can also be done continuously as needed, as in high-risk situations.

The issue with external fetal monitoring is that it is not very accurate. Since a simple movement by you or the baby can make the monitor react negatively, fetal distress can be diagnosed easily when none is present. This can lead to additional interventions, including forceps, vacuum extraction, or cesarean delivery.

Internal fetal monitoring is done when external monitoring is questioned. Since it does not rely on ultrasound to monitor your baby, it can be more accurate. This means that your water has to be broken and a thin tube with wires is inserted into your vagina and attached to your baby's scalp. This can raise the risk of infection for you and baby.

With internal fetal monitoring, your contractions may be monitored externally or with an internal uterine pressure catheter (IUPC). This is another small plastic tube that is inserted through the vagina and into the uterus, to fit just between the uterine wall and your baby. It gives very accurate measurements on how strong your contractions are. It is frequently used with Pitocin.

How do you know which monitoring method is right for you? Start by talking to your practitioner. Ask what method he uses and why, and how it can best be used for you. With the exception of the internal method, monitoring can be stopped and started at will, yours or your practitioner's.

There is an order to fetal monitoring. Low-risk women and babies start with the auscultation. If needed, you can move to external monitoring continuously, or in an emergency situation you can have the internal monitoring. The least restrictive monitoring, the more mobility you have, which means you are better able to deal with your labor. When you are able to listen to your body and choose positions that are comfortable for you, your baby tends to tolerate labor better.

If monitoring is necessary, you can still choose upright positions. Try using a birth ball next to the monitor or even a rocking chair. If you are in bed, you can still move around and assume positions, it is just more difficult.

An episiotomy is rarely necessary. And thankfully, this surgical cut is not being performed as often these days. Still, it is something you should talk to your practitioner about. Her episiotomy rate should be less than 10 percent of all labors. Ask for specifics on when this is done and how you can prevent the need for one.

Breaking your water artificially is called amniotomy. Amniotomy can be used to try and start labor or to apply internal fetal monitoring on a baby. Some practitioners believe that by breaking the water you can get the baby's head to help open the cervix. When done early in labor, however, it also increases the chance of infection and can increase the risk of prolapsed cord if the baby's head is high in your pelvis.

Your water is most likely to break at the end of labor or when you are pushing. When offered in early labor or as a matter of course, remember to ask the questions for informed consent. Why does it need to be done? What are the benefits? What are the risks? What if you do nothing? Can you do it later?

Once you agree to having your water broken, you will not be leaving the place of birth until your baby is born. This is because unlike other decisions like removing an IV and stopping a flow of medications, you cannot heal the amniotic sac. It can also be used with other interventions.

Pain Relief in Labor

Positions go a long way to helping you ease or alleviate the pain of labor. However, they are best used in combination with other methods of pain relief. There are various methods of pain relief available, many of which you will learn about in your childbirth class.

There are many forms of relaxation. You will typically think of physical relaxation, but with that comes the mental and

ASK YOUR GUIDE

Don't I want an episiotomy so I don't tear?

▶ No, you probably don't. An episiotomy can lead to excessive tearing all the way through your rectum. It is also more prone to infection and sexual problems later in life. Your vagina is meant to stretch around the baby and then go back to normal. While you may have a small tear sometimes, it is usually less extensive than an episiotomy and often requires no stitching.

emotional relaxation as well. In labor, the use of relaxation is to keep the body loose to allow the uterus to work effectively and with less pain while keeping the mind and spirit calm to prevent physical and emotional tension.

Progressive relaxation is a good first step.   You simply get comfortable in an environment you find relaxing and run through some steps that make sense to you. Many women choose to start at the top of their heads, but you can start any way you want. Pick muscles in whichever direction and begin to think of them as loose and relaxed. For example: "My head is relaxed . . . I can feel my brow loosen, my jaw slacken . . . my teeth are not clenched. I will drop my shoulders," and so on.

Another variation is tense and release relaxation. In this relaxation, you do the same thing, but rather than merely focus on relaxing a part of the body you tense it first and then consciously relax it. "I'm tightening my jaw. It feels tense. Now I will relax my jaw. Now it feels loose and open."

There are spots where many of us hold tension, like the brow, the jaw, the shoulders, and the pelvis. Having someone around who knows where you are most likely to be tense can be very helpful. I've had many a mom write me to say they felt relaxed, but their doula came up and placed a hand on their shoulders and simply said, "Relax." Then they could release just a bit more.

Practicing relaxation may seem hokey to you. It has many benefits. It can lower your stress levels in pregnancy in addition to helping you prepare for labor. There were many times I used my relaxation skills in parenting, from keeping my cool to helping a toddler relax when he was ill or during medical procedures.

It is true that the more you practice, the more easily it will come in labor. We often use excuses about not having time, or we blame our partners for not being available. But the truth is that relaxation needs to be practiced alone and with those who will be helping you.

So try to carve out five to ten minutes a day to relax, even if it's before bed. If you can't convince your husband to help, ask your doula if she can practice with you occasionally too. One mom had a great suggestion for relaxing. She said that her husband traveled a lot and couldn't always be there to practice with her. So they actually recorded a relaxation session one evening and she played it when he wasn't able to help her. I now recommend this to everyone in my childbirth classes for those days when you want to practice and he doesn't.

Breathing is necessary and helpful. I personally teach deep abdominal breathing. I think that if you can get used to taking deep breaths, you will do well in labor. This can help promote good oxygenation of you and your baby; it also has a side benefit of promoting relaxation.

Sit up straight and place your hand below your belly button. As you take a deep breath, try to breath that air all the way down to your hand. I call this breathing to your baby. Practice this several times a day in a variety of situations. It is also a really nice way to start and end relaxation sessions.

If you close your eyes while you're doing it, you can also add a bit of visualization. Some mothers tell me in class they imagine taking good air into the baby and the exhale carrying away the used air. One mom used it to visualize her baby in a head-down position. I used to just generally think a positive thought about my baby, my body, or my pregnancy. It was a nice, quiet reminder of the hard and wonderful work my body was doing in growing my baby.

Heat and cold are useful. Both techniques can be used for a variety of aches and pains in labor. Heat, like from a rice sock or warm water or clothes, is great at relieving muscle aches. It is a great way to warm cold feet or deal with pubic bone pain. Warm washcloths are also good for the perineum as the baby is crowning—they help relax the area and give mom a focus.

Cold therapy is great for more intense pains. Many moms say that cold water or an ice pack on their back really helped if they were experiencing back labor. Cool compresses during transition also can help cool a mom; try these on her head and neck.

Massage and pressure have many benefits in labor. If you enjoy a good massage, then massage in labor will probably feel very good to you. It can be used to promote relaxation and relieve pain.

Massage is used a bit differently in labor. Someone focuses on one area of the body for at least a set of contractions. This can help prevent you from becoming distracted. The touch should begin before the beginning of the contractions when possible.

Dads and doulas should always be sure to have your permission before touching you; the same goes for medical-care providers. If you do not feel like being touched, be sure to say so. Sometimes you don't want to be touched; instead, you just need to sense that those who care about you are near.

If your back is hurting, a hands-and-knees position can help alleviate the pain and give those around you a better angle to actually provide counterpressure to your back. This helps block the pain and ease the strain on your back, all while encouraging your baby to be in the best possible position in labor.

Water eases most pain in labor. The use of water in labor and birth appears to be the best form of nonmedicinal pain relief. The fancy term for this is hydrotherapy. Hydrotherapy is most commonly found in the form of a tub or a shower.

This safe, effective method of pain relief is used in many hospitals and birth centers. Some hospitals and birth centers provide tubs for use in labor, while others require that you secure the tub. Some of these tubs are specially designed to be deeper to allow more of your body to be covered in labor and to help you relax and feel buoyant. If your place of birth does not offer this, or you are planning a home birth, there are places where you can buy or rent special tubs, though this is not necessary for a water birth.

One mother wrote me to say that she had a very rough first birth and the next time she decided to try water because it seemed much more gentle. She said her labor was so calm and comfortable she thought her doctor was not being honest when he proclaimed her to be completely dilated! I used my home bathtub in labor with several of my children and it was amazing the amount of comfort I found there.

If you choose to use water in labor, find out what your practitioner says are the guidelines for use of the tub or shower. Some practitioners will only allow you to enter the tub after your labor is well established or your cervix is five centimeters dilated. The water should also be kept between 95 and 100 °F.

IV medications aren't talked about often. Before you write off these forms of medication, consider their benefits: medicinal pain relief without the same restrictions on movement and no loss of feeling or numbness. However, they can make you feel a bit like you've had some alcoholic beverage. Medications in this category include drugs like Stadol, Nubain, and Demerol.

These medications are given via your IV line or saline lock. They start taking effect within a few minutes and last for an hour or two, depending on the dose and medication given. They may be given with other medications to help prevent nausea and vomiting.

ELSEWHERE ON THE WEB

▶ Waterbirth International (www.waterbirth.org) offers information on the use of water for labor and birth along with birth stories and photos of water births. They also have a handy directory of water birth providers and ways to get a water birth tub near you.

Generally you will need to remain in bed or in a chair for a good portion of time after the administration of these medications, though with support you can move around and use different positions. The biggest side effects are itching and maternal and neonatal depressive effects, as in breathing difficulties.

Medications in this class help you to relax in between the contractions. You are less aware of the contractions and better able to cope with labor. Sometimes these medications are also used to induce sleep in very early labor or to calm nerves before a cesarean surgery.

Epidural anesthesia is one form of pain relief. This is a perfect choice for cesarean birth because it leaves the mother awake and alert and yet numb from the breasts to the legs. It has also gained popularity in the labor arena.

One in eight women suffers some sort of side effect from an epidural. Most of these are minor complications that can be reversed with some form of medical intervention. Some of the side effects that are possible with an epidural include these:

- Drop in mother's blood pressure, fetal distress
- Increased use of Pitocin
- Increased use of cesarean section or forceps
- Itching
- Nausea and vomiting
- Spinal headache
- Increase in maternal temperature leading to baby being taken to isolation
- Subtle behavioral effects on the baby, including trouble breastfeeding

This type of anesthesia is perfect for you if you want to be numb from about the breasts to at least your knees. It is also one of the choices of anesthesia for surgery. If you decide to have epidural anesthesia, you will not be allowed out of bed because you will not be able to support your body weight.

Once the decision has been made to use an epidural, you will need to talk to the anesthesiologist and sign the consent forms. She will give you an opportunity to ask any questions you have at this point.

Before you can have an epidural at some hospitals, you must have reached a certain stage of labor. This requirement may be based on how far dilated you are or simply that you are in active labor. Be sure to ask if your hospital has this requirement before you are in labor.

You will be given an IV and fluids will be run through your IV line. This is to help prevent a drop in your blood pressure, which could cause fetal distress. You will have various monitors placed on your body to measure your heart rate and blood pressure.

Typically an epidural is given while you sit upright on the bed and bend over your belly, pushing your back out for the anesthesiologist. Some moms have written to say that their husbands and support people were required to leave during the placement of the epidural. In some hospitals this is standard, while others will allow your doula to stay.

Your back will be scrubbed before anything is done. Usually you will be given an injection to numb the area where the epidural will be placed. This can sting a lot, but it is usually very brief. Then the epidural will be started.

First a needle is placed in between your vertebrae to deliver a medication around the spinal cord. Then a catheter is inserted and the needle is removed. The catheter is a small plastic tube that is

ASK YOUR GUIDE

Why do I need to know about comfort measures if I know I want an epidural?

▶ Typically, you can't have the epidural right away in labor. Most hospitals require that you do some part of labor first to prevent them from giving an epidural to someone who isn't in labor. Using these other methods for pain relief will help you through this part of labor. They may also be beneficial if your epidural doesn't work as effectively as you would like or if something happens and you can't have an epidural.

taped to your back to allow more medication to flow into the epidural space. This allows you to receive the medication constantly.

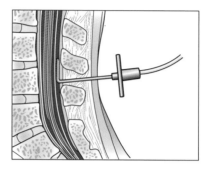

▲ Epidural insertion

After the medication is tested and you are found to be reacting well to it, you will be laid back down into your bed. Your blood pressure will be monitored every few minutes for a bit and then gradually slowed until it is just taken about every fifteen minutes, depending on your hospital.

Once you are numb, you will also get a bladder catheter since you will no longer feel the sensation to urinate. This will stay in for the duration of your labor and sometimes until a few hours after the baby is born. The bladder needs to be drained because a full bladder might prevent the baby from coming down into the pelvis.

You can now rest and sleep if your epidural is of that strength. Some moms have written that they were surprised by how much they could feel, some unpleasantly so. Be sure to talk to your anesthesiologist about how much you want to feel. Though it is important to know that you will likely have some sensation. If you still need to use comfort measures, your doula can help you find ones that are appropriate for you while laboring with an epidural.

Sometimes with an epidural your labor slows. Your doctor or midwife might recommend certain interventions to restart your labor. This might include breaking your water, the use of Pitocin, or both. Be sure to discuss the options with your practitioner before making your decision.

You will likely need help to push with the epidural. This is where having your husband and doula help you assume more upright positions is a good idea. You may also need to use more directed bearing down techniques to push effectively.

The epidural can also be used for pain relief should you need a forceps delivery or a vacuum extraction. These are used to help deliver your baby when there is an issue of time or if you are having issues with pushing. Sometimes forceps are also used to turn a baby's head that is facing the wrong direction. Be sure to ask your doctor when she would use these methods and how they differ. Should you require a cesarean, the epidural can also be used during surgery.

Once your baby is born, the epidural will also provide you with pain relief for any repair of the perineum that is needed after the birth. The catheter will usually be removed shortly after the birth is over.

Get Linked

The following links to my About.com *site will direct you to even more great information about preparing for birth, as well as some helpful photos.*

ONLINE CHILDBIRTH CLASS

Interested in learning more about childbirth? Sign up for the six-week childbirth class as an addition to your regular childbirth classes. It covers everything you need to have a great birth.

 http://about.com/pregnancy/childbirthclass

PAIN RELIEF IN LABOR

Whether you want to know about massage in labor or the use of medications like the epidural, here you'll find lots of information on all different forms of pain relief in labor, including nonmedical and medical.

 http://about.com/pregnancy/laborpainrelief

LABOR INTERVENTIONS

Interventions in labor can be frightening. Learning ahead of time about the different interventions and when and why they are used may help you reduce your fear. There is also information on avoiding the need for some interventions.

 http://about.com/pregnancy/interventions

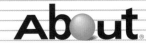

Chapter 11

Giving Birth

Labor Pain

Labor is hard work. It is a series of muscles performing actions. These actions bring about the opening of the cervix. This in turn allows passage of your baby, who will actively work with your body and your contractions to be born.

Sometimes it is best to simply look at the source of your pain. This can help you most effectively deal with the pain by addressing its causes. There are three types of pain in labor:

- Functional pain, or pain that is working toward birth
- Emotional pain, that is fear, sadness, lack of knowledge, etc.
- Abnormal pain, or pain that is not a part of the normal process

Functional pain in labor comes from different sources. Your uterine muscle tightens while working during its contractions. This causes the cervix to thin and open. Your baby is rotating and

Why does labor hurt more for some women than it does for others?

▶ Sometimes labor hurts more than what would be considered normal labor pain. This can be when there is a complication, like back labor. This means your back hurts more due to the baby being in an uncommon position. It could be from a previous injury. Sometimes additional pain in labor is caused from external sources, such as a vaginal exam or positions that are uncomfortable.

descending, causing pressure in your vagina and rectum. These are all normal processes of labor. This type of pain can be dealt with by moving around, using massage, medications, and all forms of pain relief.

Emotional pain is likely to be from causes like being worried about something in labor, lack of knowledge about what is going on, or poor communications. Sometimes this is also caused by familial strain in labor, fighting with your partner, or trying to deal with issues like your mother-in-law trying to get in the labor room. This is why surrounding yourself with supportive people like your practitioner and doula is very important. They can help you resolve these issues without taking it personally or offending your family.

The fact that there is pain in labor comes as no surprise to most women. We are not expecting a walk in the park; however, labor can often be erroneously categorized as horrible and excruciating. This is not the best way to characterize labor.

Think about hard work in your life. You probably think of being sweaty when you think of hard work, whether it's the physical work of being outside and working in your yard, or the physical work of aerobics class. Work has guttural sounds to help you put your "umpf" into it. Think of body builders lifting great loads. They sweat. They grunt. They move their bodies, all in effort. Labor is no different.

How can you incorporate those images into your idea of labor? The work of labor will probably make you work up a sweat, though not quite that of a physical laborer in the fields. You will probably make noises in labor, noises that help you do the work at hand—having a baby. You will move your body and find your way in labor, if you let your body lead.

Stages of Labor

Labor is broken down into stages to help you mentally grasp what is going on. The stages of labor have a variety of things that happen to help you give birth. Each stage is unique and requires a specific response that is best for you.

The basics of labor are simply that your cervix will dilate and efface with the help of contractions. During this period of time your baby will descend in your pelvis, measured by the station of the baby's head. When you are completely dilated and effaced and the baby is down low enough, you will feel pushing sensations to which you will respond by pushing your baby until he is born.

ASK YOUR GUIDE

How long does labor usually last?

▶ Labor usually lasts about twelve to eighteen hours for a first baby. Most of this time is spent in the earlier parts of labor. Second babies tend to come a bit faster, though any labor can have detours that make it shorter or longer. Pacing yourself in labor helps you deal with these unknowns. I was always pleasantly surprised by my shorter labors, mainly because I had told myself to prepare for the long ones. Labor is not about getting it done within a certain number of hours. It is what works best for your baby and your body.

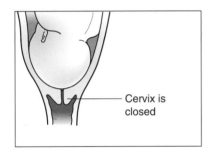

Cervix is closed

▲ Before labor

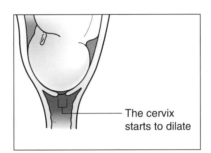

The cervix starts to dilate

▲ Early first stage

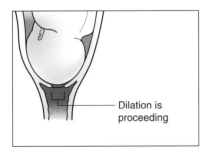

Dilation is proceeding

▲ Late first stage

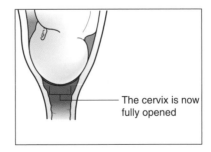

The cervix is now fully opened

▲ Fully dilated

▶ Timing contractions is an important skill. It's really very easy. You just write down the time that a contraction begins, note how long it lasts, then write down when the next contraction begins. The time from the beginning of contraction one to the beginning of contraction two is how far apart your contractions are occurring. The time from the start of the first contraction until it ends is the length of your contractions. Time a few contractions to get a general idea of where you are, and then don't do it again until there is a noticeable change.

Early labor is usually the longest part. This part of labor is where your contractions are noticeable, but light. They may be regular, but they do not usually last more than about forty-five seconds. They can be anywhere from seven to twenty minutes apart.

Typically you spend more time in the early part of labor than in any other stage of labor. The good news is that this part is very easy to deal with physically. The contractions usually don't require much, if any attention. One mom told me that her light contractions served as an early sign that she needed to finish things up because the baby would soon be here.

My advice is to have a plan as to how you intend to deal with early labor. If it is the middle of the night, go back to sleep! Get as much rest as you can, even if you're lying in bed daydreaming. During the day I'd advise you to stay busy. This can be walking, packing a bag, washing baby clothes, or going to the movies.

Early labor may not take away your appetite. Listen to your body about what it craves and when you want to eat. Most of the time your body will naturally crave a lighter fare, like bagels, fruit, crackers, tea, or broth. Avoid highly spicy or greasy foods during labor.

Several of my doula clients have spent early labor baking. Some chose to bake cookies or muffins for their midwives or the nurses at the hospital. One mom had her young children help her bake a "birth day" cake for the new baby. They were able to enjoy the cake after the birth.

You might experience any of the following in early labor:

- Light/short contractions
- Dull backache
- Loose bowels
- Excitement that the time is near
- Bloody show
- Increased vaginal discharge

Use the early part of labor to settle into labor. This is a time to have periods of rest and activity. Alternating the two will keep your mind off of labor and yet allow you to enter the next phase of labor ready to work.

Active labor is more serious.   Your contractions are closer together and probably a bit longer. They may be between five and seven minutes apart. Contractions in active labor usually last around a minute. The biggest difference in active labor is that you now need more support, and the contractions require your attention.

Your support team can help you by addressing your needs. You should remember to change positions frequently and try to go to the bathroom every hour. A full bladder will prevent your baby from descending as quickly, which can make labor longer. This is true throughout labor—change position and urinate every hour.

During this part of labor, you will want to alert your husband and doula if you have not already done so. They will help you relax during the contractions by using comfort measures. You might use massage or the birth ball. You are also able to use water now as a source of comfort.

Here are some possibilities for what you might experience in active labor:

- More intense contractions that require your attention
- Continuing bloody show and vaginal discharge
- Continuing issues from early labor

During this part of labor, you will most likely begin to use your pain relief techniques. Let comfort be your guide. While the team you have assembled is offering options to help you work with the contractions, don't fight them. But if you try a position that your body says is wrong, or you use a tool that is painful, stop using that comfort technique.

BEFORE YOUR APPOINTMENT

▶ Talk to your practitioner about when you should call. Discuss how the decision will be made for her to come to you or for you to go to the birth center or hospital. Many practitioners use the 4-1-1 plan. That's contractions four minutes apart that last at least one minute, and that go on for one hour. This is a good sign for most women that it's time to think about seeking care in labor.

Transition is the hardest but shortest part of labor. This is where you will need a lot of support from your partner and doula. They will help you stay focused and provide you with comfort measures and suggestions for positions.

The time between your contractions shrinks, and the actual length of the contraction is a bit longer. This means shorter breaks between contractions to recuperate. How you deal with this recovery time is very important to how you handle labor.

If you take the time to fully relax between your contractions, you will be more rested and better able to handle them. If you spend the break dreading the next one, you are likely to be more tense and therefore in more pain.

Here's what you might experience during transition:

○ Contractions that are close together and last about ninety seconds
○ A sense of pressure in your vagina
○ Water breaking (possibly)
○ Increased bloody show

The pushing phase is the last part of labor. Many women tell me that they were surprised by how good it felt to push. One mom said it was the physical release of being able to do something, whereas earlier in labor her body did the work and she felt it was her job to stay out of the way. Other mothers say that simply knowing it's almost over is what felt so good to them.

On average a first-time mom, without interventions, will likely push for about one and a half to two hours. During this time your baby will be making slow but steady progress downward. It will usually take you at least several contractions to get the hang of pushing.

TOOLS YOU NEED

▸ *Yoga for Pregnancy and Birth* is a great video or DVD for your collection. It includes ways to exercise during pregnancy, but I particularly like the labor section. There are specific poses shown for labor. These are easy to replicate and feel wonderful, even when you are not in labor. I highly recommend this video by *Yoga Journal* and Lamaze International.

The following list includes what you might experience during pushing:

- ○ Contractions may get slightly further apart.
- ○ Your water may break while you are pushing.
- ○ Pressure on your vagina/rectum will increase.
- ○ The sensation will be of stretching as your baby begins to crown.

Not everyone feels an urge to push.   However, if you are having a normal birth and have not chosen medication, chances are that you will feel some sort of an urge to push. Moms describe this in many ways. Some say it was simply a signal that they followed willingly. Others say that the urge to push was overwhelming and that they had no control over whether or not they pushed. If you aren't feeling an urge to push, try selecting another position to help encourage the baby in a downward movement, like squatting or standing.

Spontaneous bearing down is the act of following your body in pushing. Using this technique, you will follow the contractions and push and breath according to your body's needs. This has been shown to be the safest method for baby and mom, allowing mom to get more oxygen to her baby.

There are times when directed bearing down can be helpful. Usually this happens when a mother is experiencing a complication or has no urge to push. This is a very common procedure with an epidural since you would experience some degree of numbness. This may also be used with forceps or vacuum extraction.

If you have had an epidural, you may have issues with pushing that are different from a normal birth. Since you may not feel the urge to push, the procedure is often to have you push once

ASK YOUR GUIDE

How do they know what my cervix is doing in labor?

▶ During labor, many practitioners monitor labor's progress by the dilation of the cervix. These vaginal exams can tell you what the cervix is doing, but that might only be a part of the picture. I prefer to gauge labor's progress on the woman, her contractions, and everything in one picture. This gives a more accurate view of what is going on. The woman working really hard with her contractions is going to be giving birth much sooner than the one knitting and chatting. Avoid extra vaginal exams if labor seems to be in the same place as before.

your cervix is completely dilated. This has the potential to lead to complications with your baby's position, making it more difficult for the baby to come down or rotate correctly. Pushing too soon can make this worse.

A process called laboring down is often used. This means that rather than have you push simply because you are completely dilated, you wait until the baby has moved down on its own with the help of your uterus. Then when you push it is easier for you and your baby.

Induction

Induction of labor is done for a number of medical reasons. The American College of Obstetricians and Gynecologists (ACOG) agrees that labor should be induced only when it is dangerous for the baby to stay inside the uterus. The reasons they list for inducing labor are the following:

- Water breaks and labor does not begin
- Pregnancy has reached forty-two weeks
- Maternal hypertension
- Infection of the uterus
- Mother's health is of concern to baby, like diabetes, etc.

There are practitioners who will induce your labor for convenience reasons—theirs or yours. For no valid medical reason, this practice puts you and your baby at a greater risk, including a higher rate of intervention and cesarean section. Because of these added risks to your baby's health, think long and hard about agreeing to an induction for reasons like choosing a birthday or to avoid your practitioner's vacation.

Labor is safer when you allow it to begin on its own. Your baby is ready to be born. Your body is ready to give birth. Everything works together to help you have the safest birth possible for your baby.

The most common types of induction include these:

- Medications (orally, vaginally, or IV)
- Rupturing the membranes (amniotic sac)
- A combination of methods

Sometimes it's hard to know if an induction is necessary. Perhaps you've been told that you are expecting a large baby and that you should consider induction. ACOG does not believe that you need to schedule an induction for this reason. They cite that prediction methods including ultrasound are often considerably off. This makes it hard to say who really has a big baby and who doesn't. It also can't tell you how your body or your baby's body will react to labor. Remember your pelvis is not a stationary object. As you move and assume positions, your pelvis will move and give to allow your baby safe passage. In turn, your baby's head is designed to move and fit through your pelvis, too. It's your body's perfect plan for labor. Any interference with this plan can put your baby and you at risk.

Ask yourself why your labor needs to be induced. Is there a clear medical reason? If not, be sure to find out why induction is being proposed. Many practices will induce labor for nonmedical reasons. This is not a good reason to subject you or your baby to these added risks.

Cesarean Section

The cesarean section or c-section rate is almost a third of all births. This is well above what the World Health Organization (WHO) says it should be. They argue that even high-risk centers should have a 15-percent cesarean rate and that low-risk centers and such should aim for 5.

So why are so many women giving birth by cesarean? The answer is not that your body will fail you, but that the medical

WHAT'S HOT

▶ I get lots of e-mail about how to know when your water has broken. Typically speaking, your water won't break until you're pretty far into labor. About 75 percent of all women won't experience this until transition. If you're unsure, try this tip: Put on a clean sanitary pad and lie down for about thirty minutes. If there is a gush of fluid when you sit up, chances are your water has broken.

system will likely be the source of the failure. With the added interventions and legal risks, many women are having interventions that increase the surgical birth rate. Practitioners are also coercing women into believing that cesareans are the best choice for them or their babies.

Cesarean surgery has been designed to protect the life and health of you and your baby. This is still true. The problem is not that there is something wrong with this surgery, but that it is over-used in nonproblematic, normal, healthy women and their babies. Medical reasons for cesarean section include the following:

- Placenta abruption
- Cord prolapse
- Placenta previa
- Malpresentation of the baby (transverse lie, certain breeches, etc.)
- Maternal disease, like active herpes, diabetes, etc.
- Congenital anomalies of the baby made worse by vaginal birth
- Higher-order multiples
- Fetal distress
- Lack of labor progress

How can you prevent an unnecessary cesarean? Find a practitioner who believes that birth is a normal process. Ask what the primary cesarean rate is in their practice and for themselves. Ask when they feel interventions like induction and cesarean should be used.

Asking these questions should give you an idea of their philosophy of birth. If the practitioner has a philosophy of birth as normal and uses surgery for only the rarest of emergencies, and you feel comfortable, then you have a good match.

ELSEWHERE ON THE WEB

▶ Trying to sort out the mixed messages that society sends about induction? The Lamaze Institute for Normal Birth has a paper plainly stating the benefits and risks of induction in a medically safe and sound but understandable format. Check it out at www.lamaze.org/institute/carepractices/LaborBegins.asp.

Sometimes choosing a cesarean birth is the best thing for you and your baby. Making this decision may be easy, or it may be difficult. Sometimes you may know before your due date that a cesarean birth is the safest way for your baby to be born, for example, if you have a placenta previa. This is called a scheduled cesarean. An unscheduled cesarean is when you are in labor and the need for a cesarean arises, but is not an emergency. An emergency cesarean is done within several minutes of the decision and is frequently done with general anesthesia.

The cesarean section usually takes just under an hour to perform. Just before surgery, you will have a series of tasks performed. You will take an antacid, either orally or by IV. You will also have the upper portion of your pubic hair shaved. Several monitors will also be placed on your torso, arm, and finger to monitor various bodily functions like blood pressure and heart rate.

If you did not previously have a spinal or epidural during labor, you will usually have one administered in the operating room. You will also need a bladder catheter that will stay in for about twenty-four hours. This is to help prevent your bladder from being nicked or cut during the surgery and to drain the bladder before, during, and after your surgery.

The surgical team will drape your body with coverings and blankets. They will also lift a small drape between your head and your abdomen to prevent you from contaminating the sterile field. You may have your legs strapped down, to prevent you from falling off the table since your body is numb.

You will have oxygen either by mask or with tubing in your nostrils. They may also strap your hands down. Your husband or other support person will be able to sit by your head to talk to you. He will also have to wear surgical scrubs into the operating room.

Usually there will be many people in the room. This comes as a shock to many people when they have a cesarean. People in the room when you have a cesarean may include the following:

- A support person or two (husband, doula, etc.)
- Your doctor
- Assistant surgeon
- Anesthesiologist
- Scrub nurse or scrub tech
- Nursery nurse
- Neonatologist or pediatrician
- Other support personnel as needed

Once the surgery is started, the birth usually happens very quickly, in about five to ten minutes. The incision on your abdomen is usually a "bikini" incision, done horizontally just above your pubic hairline. In some emergencies or situations a vertical or "classical" incision may be made under your belly button.

During the surgery you should not feel any sharp pain. If you do, say something to the anesthesiologist, who will be sitting right near your head. You may feel pressure and what they commonly refer to as pushes, pulls, and tugs.

Once the surgeon has cut through all the layers to get to the uterus, the amniotic sac is punctured. The baby is then lifted out of the pelvis and through the incision. Your baby's position will determine if he is born head first or bottom first. You can watch this with a mirror, if you desire. This is safe because all you will see will be your baby's head.

After that, the baby will be shown to you briefly over the drape and then taken to a warmer for evaluation. Here they will weigh and measure your baby. He may have vitamin K injections or other vaccinations you have agreed to in your admission paperwork.

▶ While the baby is at the warming table, you may wish to have your husband go over and hold the baby's hand and talk to him. Usually you can take photos now as well. These are great to have for later, because you can't be right next to the baby at this time. Hopefully after a brief visit at the warmer, the baby can be bundled up and brought to you. Remind your husband to walk carefully to your head. If he is squeamish, he won't want to look around the room.

They will listen to the baby's heart and lungs and treat him for any issues with breathing as needed. It is not uncommon for babies to receive a bit of oxygen at first. They may also do additional suctioning as necessary.

The rest of the surgery will take about thirty or forty more minutes. This is because the removal of the placenta and the repair of the layers of the incision take more time than making the incision. The suture material used inside your body is made to absorb into your body and does not need to be removed. The outside incision is closed with either medical-grade staples or regular stitching material. The decision of which to use is based on your surgeon's preference as well as your body type.

After the surgery you will spend about an hour to an hour and a half in a recovery room. While in this area, you can usually have your baby and the same support people that were in the operating room with you. You will be monitored for postsurgical complications. You will also have your postpartum bleeding and your pain monitored.

Initially, you will use the spinal or epidural as pain relief after the surgery. Most surgeons can place something in the spinal or epidural to help relieve pain but not numb the area. This medication can last sixteen to twenty-four hours. On top of this medication, you can also have oral or IV medications for pain relief. You may also be prescribed over-the-counter medications in addition to the heavy-duty pain medications.

While in the recovery room you should feel free to get to know your baby. Breastfeeding is highly encouraged. Breastfeeding will provide both you and the baby with benefits at this point.

After the initial postpartum period in the recovery room, you will move to the postpartum floor. You will stay in this area for the next three or four days. Here you will receive postsurgical as well as postpartum care.

ELSEWHERE ON THE WEB

▶ Childbirth Connection has a great resource on cesarean section and vaginal birth after cesarean, particularly when it comes to assistance in making decisions. You can read the latest information on the safety of all of your options for you and your baby. Plus, you'll find great decision-making tools that give you facts while busting myths of things you may have heard that might not be true. Visit the Web site at www.childbirthconnection.org.

Cesarean surgery can be family centered. There are things that you can ask for that will help make your cesarean surgery have more of a birth feel to it. Some ideas include the following:

- Ask to have your hand(s) untied to touch the baby immediately.
- Use a mirror to watch the birth.
- Have the main operating room lights dimmed and use a spotlight for the surgical field.
- Have your husband or other support person announce the sex of the baby.
- Breastfeed as the surgery is being finished with the help of your doula.
- Play music in the operating room.

Having a cesarean section does not mean that you have to give up everything that you wanted about postpartum. While you will be in the hospital longer and you will be recovering from surgery, there is nothing to stop you from breastfeeding immediately or rooming-in. You may need help to make these things happen.

Vaginal Birth After Cesarean (VBAC)

Vaginal birth after cesarean (VBAC) is an option for most women who have had a previous cesarean birth. The decision to have a vaginal birth after a previous cesarean is not always an easy one. Medical studies show that when given the opportunity, you have a greater than 80-percent chance of having a successful vaginal birth.

There are things you need to know to make a decision about whether you wish to have a VBAC or whether you want to repeat a cesarean surgery for your next baby. In addition to being highly likely that you will have a vaginal birth, VBAC is incredibly safe. Here are some of the benefits of a VBAC:

- Fewer breathing problems in newborns
- Lower risk of infection
- Fewer problems in future pregnancies

The biggest fear with a VBAC is the slight risk that the previous scar may open during labor. This risk is less than 1 percent.

There are risks to repeated cesareans. Whenever you do surgery, there are risks involved. The risk of infection and injury to the mother's bladder is increased. There are also risks to the baby, like being born early or having breathing difficulties, which may necessitate a longer stay in the hospital or even more intensive care.

Laboring as a VBAC is different. Currently, the majority of women having a VBAC do so with constant fetal monitoring. There is likely to be more intervention from some practitioners, so be sure to ask why a procedure is being proposed so that you can figure out if it's normal for every laboring mom or simply because you are a VBAC.

Trigger points can happen in labor. This is where you have a memory from your previous birth that can be worrisome or make you feel like you can't have a vaginal birth. My sister had a cesarean for her first baby, and for her second baby she planned a VBAC. She said that simply hearing that she was three centimeters dilated really brought her first labor back. She said she felt like she was going to get stuck again. She was glad to hear that she had changed and was then six centimeters and had a great VBAC experience.

ELSEWHERE ON THE WEB

▶ Finding solid information about safe VBAC, practitioners who are experienced in VBAC, and a good support network can be difficult. Save yourself the trouble of looking around. Visit this site for fact-filled papers, local resources, and support in the way of stories from other families, and interactive support from e-mail and chat groups: www.ican-online.org.

Get Linked

There is so much to know about giving birth. How do you even start to fill your mind with the knowledge? Below are some links that will help you wrap your mind around the work and reward of labor.

VAGINAL BIRTH AFTER CESAREAN (VBAC)

Planning a vaginal birth after a cesarean requires thought and support. Learn how to ask the right questions to find a supportive and knowledgeable practitioner in your area as well as find the mental and emotional support you need to have your successful VBAC.

 http://about.com/pregnancy/vbac

CESAREAN PREVENTION

Interested in learning how you can prevent a cesarean section? There are ways to lower your risk of having surgery without compromising the health of your baby.

 http://about.com/pregnancy/preventcsection

CESAREAN BIRTH

These cesarean birth links include birth stories, photo galleries, and family-centered cesarean information, as well as a cesarean birth plan. Also included is information on cesarean recovery and breastfeeding after a cesarean.

 http://about.com/pregnancy/cesarean

Chapter 12

Breastfeeding

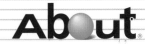
Educating Your Family for Success

Breastfeeding is something you can do. It is much harder to do when you are trying to nurse your baby in a vacuum. Filling your environment with knowledgeable and supportive people can only help you as you nourish your family.

Start with the basics of breastfeeding for your family. Talk about how breastfeeding benefits the baby, you, and even the family. Here are just a few of the many reasons breastfeeding is best for your baby and your family:

- The American Academy of Pediatrics (AAP) recommends it, as do many medical organizations.
- Breastfed babies have higher IQs.
- Breast milk is easily digestible and less likely to cause reflux or upset stomach.
- It helps mom's uterus shrink and burns extra calories.

- Breastfed babies have fewer ear infections as well as upper respiratory infections.
- It is much easier than other alternatives.
- You're less likely to get breast cancer.
- Baby is likely to develop fewer allergies.

ELSEWHERE ON THE WEB

▶ The benefits of breastfeeding are numerous; I could fill a whole book with the great reasons that breastfeeding is best for your baby, you, and your family. I'll just stick with the handful above, but check out this well organized list of 101 Reasons to Breastfeed (www.promom.org/101). It's perfect for learning about breastfeeding for you or for reluctant family members.

Consider taking those who will be helping you after the baby is born to a breastfeeding class or support group. This can help them see that someone else has the same beliefs as you do and is willing to help them help you. Sometimes support can be hindered simply because your husband, mother, sister, or friend doesn't know enough about breastfeeding to be helpful.

A class is the perfect answer to help your supporters to get that knowledge. When picking a class, try to think of the person you are taking with you. Is it someone who wants to hear from others mothers who are actually breastfeeding? Or does she prefer authority figures, such as the doctors at a local hospital, to tell her why they recommend breastfeeding?

You will get well-meaning but inaccurate advice. This advice can come from everyone from your postpartum nurse to your mother-in-law. This makes the first few days and weeks very hard, particularly if this is your first baby, because you don't know to whom you should listen.

When trying to find out whether or not you should listen to advice, remember that the best advice will come from other mothers who have successfully nursed their children. Often the training in medical and nursing school is not adequate for helping new mothers learn to nurse effectively. Many medical groups now employ their own lactation consultants.

Asking the wrong person can mean getting bad advice, but worse than getting bad advice is getting conflicting advice. Many a mom has told me that she would ask a simple question about nursing her baby and get a different response from every nursing shift. So when in doubt, find out who really knows. Ask some simple questions, like these:

- Did you breastfeed your children? If so, for how long?
- Are you a lactation consultant?
- What specifically is your training in breastfeeding?

If you are afraid you really are having trouble finding a knowledgeable person, call someone like a private lactation consultant or a support group of peer counselors, like La Leche League, for advice and support. Many will make hospital and house calls. Need a referral? Ask friends and others who have successfully nursed for recommendations.

Preparation will help ease problems. By learning the basics before your baby is born, you will increase your comfort level with breastfeeding and have some of the basic questions answered. This knowledge comes from many different sources, including attending breastfeeding classes, reading breastfeeding books, or attending breastfeeding support groups or peer counseling sessions.

The more knowledge you have going into breastfeeding, the better off you are when your baby arrives. You will feel confident in the process and know what to expect. You will understand how your body works to make milk for your baby and how your baby nurses to get that milk.

There are times when you will need help when breastfeeding. Sometimes you will need emotional support, which may revolve around new motherhood in general, breastfeeding

ASK YOUR GUIDE

Is there someone at the hospital to help me learn to nurse?

▶ Most of the time there is a lactation consultant available. Be sure when you take a tour of your place of birth that you ask them what hours a lactation consultant works, so you'll be sure to get her in to see you. The problem can sometimes be that you have your baby and are out of the hospital before she's back on duty. Find out if you can get a private lactation consultant or if you can come back to the hospital after birth for help and advice.

ELSEWHERE ON THE WEB

▶ La Leche League (www
.lalecheleague.org) offers
free classes on breastfeeding
every month in most cit-
ies around the world. Topics include the benefits of
breastfeeding, first feedings,
common issues with breastfeeding, starting solid foods,
and weaning from the breast.
These can be great sources
of information for you as well
as other family members.
Many moms tell me they go
for the information, but they
come back for the support.

specifically, or any combination of issues. This is for all mothers and
not just first-time mothers.

There are also times when you will need support for physical
issues with breastfeeding. This might be because of a problem or
from questions that you have about breastfeeding. An example
might be problems with your baby's latch that are causing you
pain or questions about how to deal with breastfeeding issues,
like how long to nurse or if your baby needs anything else.

Most of the time the support you need is brief in nature. It
might be a quick question or a fast visit to help make a slight adjustment to how you hold your baby. Knowing where to go or whom
to call can really help when the situation arises, so be prepared!

Ongoing support is nice for all mothers. This is usually
in the form of answering questions and simply being around like-
minded individuals. You can sometimes see this by way of new
mothers groups that are informal, like neighborhood groups. You
may also see more formal organizations aimed at new mothers,
like Mothers of Twins Clubs or local Mother's Centers.

There are also breastfeeding specific groups that gather for
that support. La Leche League International (LLLI) is probably the
biggest and best known of these types of groups available. They
hold monthly gatherings in every state and many countries around
the world. Some communities have more than one meeting group.
These groups vary by time and location, though the content is
much the same. There are also other peer breastfeeding support
groups available.

The ongoing lessons at La Leche and other peer counseling
centers are centered upon breastfeeding. For example, you might
learn about the benefits of breastfeeding or how and when to
start solid foods and when to wean your baby. But the way the
meetings work varies by the leader in charge and the mothers who

attend. As with any group dynamics situation, find the group that works best with your needs, be it location or philosophy. The goal of these groups is to reach out to all nursing mothers, no matter what their goals are in terms of breastfeeding.

Basic Breastfeeding Positioning

Positioning for breastfeeding goes hand in hand with a good latch. You cannot have one without the other. In fact, a large portion of what is wrong with many latches is the position.

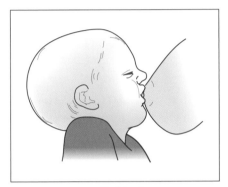

▲ Bad latch

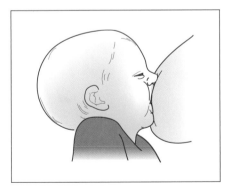

▲ Good latch

ELSEWHERE ON THE WEB

▶ A lactation consultant (International Board Certified Lactation Consultant [IBCLC]) is someone trained in breastfeeding support and management. When experiencing breastfeeding issues, I highly recommend that you find one of these handy helpers to assist you in breastfeeding. As with any support professional, be sure your personalities and goals match before agreeing to work together. You might find one at your local hospital or birth center, or you can search the Web at www.iblce.org.

The best positions for mothers and babies are those in which mom is comfortable and relaxed. You should also be well supported by your chair or seat, with or without pillows. I would recommend finding a position to start with and to learn breastfeeding from there.

The cradle hold is a common one to see mothers using in the first feedings. The key to this position is to make sure that you and the baby are belly to belly and that she is not facing upward. You should also make sure that your baby is not lying at an angle and is perfectly horizontal to your body. These will maximize a good latch.

If you are feeding from the right breast, you will cradle the baby's head on the forearm portion of your right arm, just before the crook. Use your left hand to form a C shape to hold the breast. This gives you control over the breast without your hand getting in your baby's way.

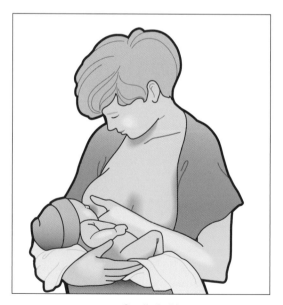

▲ Cradle hold

The cross-cradle hold is very similar. If you were feeding from the right breast, the baby would lie his body on your left arm, using your left hand at the back of his head and neck to help control where he puts his head. You would then form your right hand in the C position to maneuver your right breast. I actually prefer the cross-cradle hold for learning to breastfeed.

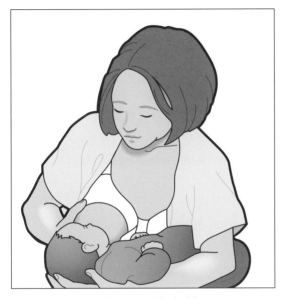

▲ Cross-cradle hold

WHAT'S HOT

▶ Well-meaning friends and relatives may try to tell you that the breastfed baby needs water. A breastfed baby does not need anything other than mother's milk until at least six months of age, and that includes water. Your breast milk has everything to nourish and hydrate your baby. Giving your baby water can actually be harmful, so avoid supplementing your breastfeeding sessions with water.

As your baby gets older you will be able to branch out into many different nursing positions. Do not feel constrained by what anyone or any book tells you is the one perfect position to nurse. It really is about finding a good fit for you and your baby.

Some positions are more comfortable after a cesarean birth. One of the most commonly talked about is the football or clutch hold. This allows you to nurse comfortably, without placing the baby on or near your abdomen.

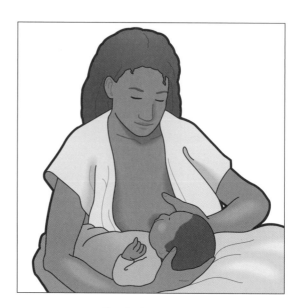

▲ Football or clutch hold

In an upright position, choose a side to nurse. Hold the baby, bottom first into your side with that same arm. If your baby is very long or large, the baby's legs may go up the back of your bed or chair, or wrap around your back, whatever is comfortable for you.

Use your opposite hand to form a C and maneuver the breast. So if your left arm is holding the baby and managing his head, much like in the cross-cradle hold, your right hand would hold the left breast. This allows you a good look at the latch as well as protecting your incision, which will be sore for some time.

A side-lying breastfeeding position is also good if you have had abdominal surgery. This one takes a bit more skill in my opinion, but it should be given a try, because practice will make it easier. Choose either side to lie on and put a pillow behind your back for support.

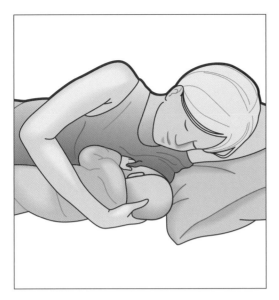

▲ Side-lying position

Turn your baby onto her side as well, facing your body. Her mouth should be slightly lower than your breast (think nipple to nose) so that when she opens wide your nipple points to the roof of her mouth to aid in a better latch. Once baby is latched, settle in.

You may prefer to lie all the way down with your bottom arm extended or wrapped under your head. Other mothers tell me they prefer to lift up on the bottom elbow. It is whatever is most comfortable for you.

Getting Started with Nursing

Breast milk is made on the principle of demand and supply. Your baby demands milk by nursing and your body supplies it. It really is that simple.

TOOLS YOU NEED

▶ A breastfeeding pillow can be a handy thing to have around, particularly early on in your breastfeeding relationship. I liked it because it helped me get a grasp on my tiny baby while trying to learn to hold my breast and position the baby as well. It also provided me with support to my arms and back so I could relax while nursing. Later I used the pillow for playing with the baby, like tummy time. They even make breastfeeding pillows for twins.

There are two things that help this process along smoothly. One is a good latch of the baby to the breast, which is aided by the other thing, a good position. A good latch is obtained by having the baby open his mouth wide, like you would do if you were eating a large sandwich, and aiming your nipple toward the roof of his mouth. Pull the baby quickly toward your breast; do not go to the baby with the breast, as this will cause you back strain.

You can express a drop or two of milk before trying to get your baby to latch on your breast. The smell and taste may entice your baby to open wide to get a good latch. But be sure to remove your hands from the areola while trying to latch your baby on.

He should take a good portion of the areola tissue in his mouth. His mouth should open wide with his lips flanged around your breast. When he nurses, you should not feel pain. If you feel pain, you need to break the suction by placing a finger in the side of his mouth. Keep relatching him until the sucking portion of feeding does not hurt. Positioning the baby is important to a good, pain-free latch as well getting the baby the milk he needs.

Good positioning is when the baby's head is aligned with his body, and his face, chin, stomach, and legs are facing your body. His head should not be twisting or turning, nor facing up. I like to say belly to belly and chin to breast. When a baby is twisted or even has his head slightly turned, it makes getting the milk out of the breast very difficult for him.

You will know when your baby is latched well when the following things happen:

- His ears wiggle.
- After ten sucks, you hear swallowing.
- You see the pink part of his lips.
- There are no clicking or smacking sounds.
- Milk does not leak from his mouth at the corners.

Your first feeding should happen within minutes of birth.
This is according to the American Academy of Pediatrics (AAP). The first few hours of your baby's life has him in the perfect state to learn to nurse. He is in a great quiet, alert state and ready and willing to nurse.

Simply have him come immediately from being born to your abdomen and then to your breast. Many mothers say that they didn't have to do anything, that the baby knew exactly what to do. Other moms say that it took a few minutes and some nudging before the baby had a good latch. Some of this will depend on the birth and the baby, but either scenario is fine.

Suckling at the breast has a very good and calming effect on the baby after birth. It also helps your uterus contract back down. This decreases the bleeding you will have after birth.

Your baby may lie on your abdomen skin-to-skin for quite awhile. This is the warmest place for him. Be sure to use a dry towel or blanket to cover both of you. This maintains the radiant heat that you produce. You may also wish to cover his head with a small cap or hat.

The skin-to-skin contact will also help him nurse. He will be free to smell or lick at the nipple and finally latch on. You can help your baby by placing him very close to the nipple.

This can be a very sweet and lovely time. It need not be interrupted by the hospital or birth center except in the case of true medical emergencies, like if your baby were not breathing. Most other tasks that hospitals need to do can wait or be done while the baby is on your body.

I would recommend that you talk to your doctor or midwife prior to the birth about this uninterrupted time. You may be asked to get this okayed by a pediatrician or other health-care provider on your birth plan. It is not usually a problem as the vast majority of babies have no difficulties.

The first milk your baby gets is called colostrum. Colostrum is high in antibodies and has a laxative effect on your baby. This helps your baby more quickly pass the meconium that lines his intestines. This can also help to prevent or lessen the effects of jaundice in the newborn period.

As you get to know your baby, it will be very easy to learn his hunger cues. Remember, the sooner you feed your baby the easier it will be to nurse because you will not have to calm your baby first. Here are the most common cues listed in relative order of when they occur:

- Opening and closing his mouth
- Smacking lips together
- Sucking on anything (lips, tongue, hands, toys, or clothes)
- Rooting on anyone
- Trying to position himself to nurse
- Being fidgety
- Breathing rapidly
- Fussing
- Moving his head frantically
- Crying

Feeding in the first weeks is an adjustment period. You will be learning your baby just as your baby is learning you. You will want to nurse your baby about ten to twelve times a day during the first week to help establish a good milk supply. You can feed your baby too little, but you cannot feed your baby too often. The more your baby nurses, the better milk supply you build.

Your milk is created on a demand-and-supply scenario. Your baby demands milk. Your body supplies it. Your milk usually comes in between day three and day seven.

These first feedings will not be evenly spaced. Do not worry about a pattern of nursing in the first weeks. If your baby is sleeping, remember to wake him to nurse every two hours during the day. This will help him have longer periods of sleep at night. If your baby is sleeping longer than four hours at night, you should wake him this often to eat. This will prevent drops in your milk supply.

After that first week, you will probably feed your baby eight to twelve times a day, depending on your baby's needs. Some babies like to cluster feed around their fussy time of day. This means that they may nurse every hour for three or four hours for a short period and then have a long sleep. This is normal and is not a sign of a problem. Remember, your baby cannot read a clock.

You will know how long to feed your baby per breast. Once the baby is latched onto the breast you should allow him to nurse until he stops. This may be a few minutes or longer. Once he has finished one side, offer the second breast. To help facilitate an even supply, be sure to start on the breast you left off on at the last feeding. So if you start nursing on the right and end on the left breast, the next feeding should begin with the left breast. I use a plastic bracelet on my hand that I move back and forth to remind me where to start. A couple of mothers told me that they used a safety pin on their bra to indicate which breast to offer first.

Learn to tell when your baby is full. Your baby may fall asleep at the breast. He may also pull away from the breast to indicate that he is finished with a feeding.

You should also learn to tell if your baby is eating enough. The number of bowel movements your baby has a day can vary widely. Needless to say, during the first few days, as your baby is clearing

WHAT'S HOT

▶ It is normal for your baby to lose up to 7 to 10 percent of his birth weight in the first few days of life. This is not a cause for alarm, nor is it a sign that you should supplement your breastfeeding. I would encourage you to take your baby for a weight check by the lactation consultant or your pediatrician at the end of the first week of life to help you ensure that your baby is on the right track.

the meconium out of his system, he will have a bowel movement once or more a day. By the time your baby is three to six weeks old, his stooling pattern may be once every day or once every week. Both are fine. The definition of a bowel movement is only the size of a quarter. It is also not uncommon for some babies to have a bowel movement at every feeding. By day four, as the meconium is gone, the bowel movements should be seedy and yellow in color. They are also more runny than an adult bowel movement. This is not diarrhea.

Your baby should urinate six to eight times a day. In disposable diapers, this can be hard to see. I would recommend that you put a tissue in the diaper to help you ascertain if your baby has urinated. Be sure to check your baby's diaper often, so that you don't miss a wet diaper. Typically, cloth diapers will be wet closer to eight and disposable diapers closer to six times a day.

You cannot generally tell how well nursing is going by how often your baby wants to eat. Nor can you really tell by how full your breasts are or aren't, particularly after a while. Watching the number of nursing sessions per day, the wet and dirty diapers, as well as baby's weight gain are the best indicators of a nursing baby doing well.

Some babies have special breastfeeding needs. If you have a baby who was born early or needs special care because of a problem like Down syndrome or a cleft lip and/or palate, be sure to seek support from a knowledgeable lactation consultant. Even babies with problems can nurse well with the proper support.

If your baby has problems nursing, be sure to get help with your milk supply. This may involve both breastfeeding and pumping milk for your baby. But the sickest of babies especially need breast milk to help them heal, and grow more quickly and grow stronger.

Common Issues with Breastfeeding

Breastfeeding often goes without problems, particularly if mom and baby were given early and ample time at birth to begin breast-feeding. Some interventions in labor can also be a cause of early breastfeeding issues, but these can be worked through quickly with a bit of patience and knowledge.

Sore nipples can happen. Usually sore nipples are caused by a bad latch. Be sure that you follow the guidelines for a good latch and are using a good position. Have a professional watch you nurse. If you have pain, something is not right.

Breastfeeding can feel strange if you have never nursed. You should feel tugging and pulling. You might even feel a tingling as your milk lets down. But pain is not normal and needs to be evaluated by someone experienced.

The sooner you get help, the better off you will be. Not correcting an improper latch can lead to severe problems like cracked and bleeding nipples. Early and frequent help can help prevent this more serious complication.

Engorgement of the breasts hurts. If your breasts make too much milk, you may suffer from engorgement. This makes your breasts hurt, and it makes it harder for your baby to breast-feed well. If you take warm compresses to your breasts before nursing, it can soften the nipple enough for your baby to be able to latch on. I used newborn diapers filled with water as hot as I could stand as compresses. They held the water without dripping and I didn't have to take a shower all the time.

You can also add a bit of massage to this to help move the milk. Using a breast pump also works, though you want to only pump enough to relieve the pressure. Too much pumping can actually cause the milk production to increase.

ELSEWHERE ON THE WEB

▶ I love www.kellymom.com. It is a great resource for nursing moms everywhere, no matter what your nursing or pumping question, with super videos and pictures, as well as practical advice. I have yet to look up a topic that is not covered. I love the down-to-earth nature of the advice and how it is presented. It is also very easy to find what you are looking for on this site.

Once the nipple is softer, baby is usually able to latch on without issue. Then you can allow the baby to regulate how much milk she needs at any given time. By allowing the baby to nurse often, particularly in the first weeks of life, you can be assured that you will establish the right amount of milk for your baby.

Growth spurts make babies hungry.   During these growth spurts, your baby may nurse more often as a way to tell your body to make more milk. These increased feedings often last for a few days, in order to build a bigger milk supply. Then your baby goes back to his normal nursing pattern.

You can expect growth spurts when your baby reaches between seven and ten days of age, between two and three weeks, and between four and six weeks. Do not panic about these increased feedings during this time. It is not a permanent thing and will subside as soon as your body responds with more milk.

Your body can supply enough milk.   Occasionally there may be problems with a small supply if you or your baby has been ill or if there was not an adequate amount of nursing in the beginning. These supply problems can be overcome with proper care and some time.

The first step is to offer the baby your breast more frequently. This can solve many cases of low supply and very quickly. Usually you will be asked to pump your breasts to increase your supply if simply increasing baby's nursing time alone is not effective. Be sure to follow the advice of a lactation professional as supplementing at this time can be detrimental to your milk supply if done incorrectly.

Jaundice can be normal.   In the first few days of your baby's life, he may turn slightly yellow due to a lack of bilirubin breaking down in his body. Breast milk actually helps jaundice resolve more

▶ Check for inverted nipples prior to your next appointment by depressing the widest part of the areola and letting go. If your nipple goes inside the breast tissue, you may have inverted nipples. This does not mean that breastfeeding is not possible, it simply means that you may need to do some exercises or wear breast shells to help evert your nipples. The best way to get your nipple everted is by letting your baby latch on. Talk to your practitioner at the next appointment about how to best treat this, or ask to seek care from a lactation consultant.

quickly because it helps expel meconium by acting like a laxative. If your baby has jaundice, you should still be allowed to nurse, no matter what the cause.

Pumping and Alternatives to Breastfeeding

Sometimes pumping your breast milk is necessary for you or your baby. This can be because of extended separation or illness in your baby. What pump you choose will reflect your needs, how much milk you need, and how long you intend to pump.

Hospital pumps are designed for heavy-duty use. One of the biggest issues with using a breast pump is to determine why you are using it. A good, solid, multi-user pump is designed to initiate and maintain a milk supply. This makes it the perfect choice for when you need to pump right from the beginning of your baby's life. Such pumps are all capable of doing double pumping.

Large electric pumps are great for working mothers. Even the most expensive and nice breast pump that is only for a single user is not designed to initiate a supply. These pumps are designed to maintain your supply. They do so very nicely. The more times a day you pump, the better they are for your purpose. These breast pumps may be single or double pumps.

Occasional-use pumps are nice to have around. Hand pumps or small electric pumps do not maintain a supply. Nor do they initiate one. These pumps are used mainly for an occasional time away from your baby and are usually single pumps only.

There are alternatives to bottles. If your baby needs to be fed pumped breast milk or artificial baby milk, avoid bottles for a minimum of six to eight weeks or until breastfeeding is well

TOOLS YOU NEED

▶ A blanket comes in handy when trying to nurse a flailing baby. Simply use the blanket to help pin your baby's arms at her sides. This keeps her from batting at your breasts or pulling herself off a great latch. You can use any swaddle wrap that works best for you, or you can use one of the blankets that are specifically made for swaddling. If the temperature is excessively warm, consider using a folded blanket just to hold her arms closer to her body.

established. You should also avoid these if you have a baby who has latch issues. Some alternatives to baby bottles include:

- Special cups
- Hazelbaker finger feeder
- Supplemental nursing system (SNS)
- Syringe

These means of feeding your baby preserve the proper suckling and latching instinct. They do not give your baby an easy way out. However, you should be shown how to use them to your advantage and how to use them correctly to help you correct whatever problem you are having. While there is no harm in long-term use, it is easier to get the baby back to the breast.

Once breastfeeding is well established and supply issues have been dealt with, you may choose to use baby bottles to feed your baby expressed breast milk. Try different bottles to find the best for your baby. Be sure to always use slow-flow nipples, no matter how old your baby is, when using the baby bottle.

Some mothers pump breast milk. This may be done because you work away from your baby, because you choose to feed your baby breast milk without nursing, or because you or your baby has a medical problem requiring you to pump your breast milk. There are many reasons that mothers choose to pump. If you are choosing to pump because of medical reasons, be sure to seek the advice of your lactation consultant to help you achieve whatever your goal is for pumping. This may be to relieve engorgement or to build your milk supply. Pumping for either of these reasons would be done very differently.

When trying to increase your supply, it is best to offer the baby your breast first. After the baby is satisfied, then use the breast

What if I decide not to or can't breastfeed?

▸ Some mothers choose to exclusively feed their babies breast milk but can't or choose not to breastfeed. If this is your situation, it is important that you begin pumping within a few hours of birth and pump around the clock, just as a new baby would nurse. I wound up pumping like this for my twins for the first three months of their lives. Eventually they went to the breast and I was able to stop pumping breast milk to feed them, except when I was away from them for extended periods of time. Many moms set one year as their goal to stop pumping since it is the minimum amount of time recommended by the American Academy of Pediatrics.

pump. Save whatever you pump to feed your baby at a later time or to finish the feeding. Remember that the more stimulation your breast gets, either through your baby or your breast pump, the more milk you will make.

If you are pumping because you will be working away from your baby, you should plan to replace normal feedings with pumping sessions. After you have been pumping for a while, you may find that you are able to pump enough during fewer sessions if you double pump, and still make enough milk to cover more than one feeding per pumping session.

Supplements are rarely needed. If supplementation is suggested by your breastfeeding professional, be sure to find out why and what you can do to minimize the need for supplements. Consider pumping milk to supplement your breastfeeding.

According to the World Health Organization (WHO), your breast milk is best, followed by your expressed breast milk. Then the next best option is the expressed breast milk of another mother. This can be obtained from a breast milk bank. This milk is pasteurized and safe. Insurance companies may cover these costs.

According to WHO, the last option is artificial baby milk (ABM). Since there are risks to using ABM, you will want to work with the lactation specialist to decide which is right for your baby. Unless you are prescribed a particular, specialty ABM, your insurance is not usually willing to cover this increased cost. Be sure to ask at the hospital or ask the pharmacist.

Normally, building your milk supply is all that is needed, and the supplementation can be stopped. It usually takes a week or so to build your supply, though you will see improvements within a few days. If you choose to use supplementation long term, discuss the health ramifications with your pediatrician.

WHAT'S HOT

▶ Though you may be told that solids will reduce the number of spitting-up episodes or that solids will help your baby sleep through the night, the truth of the matter is that starting solids should not happen prior to about six months of age. This is because your baby's body is not physically ready for anything but breast milk prior to this age. In addition to hazards like an increase in allergies, you run the risk of causing your baby to choke because he isn't ready for solids physically. Solids, including runny cereal, should never be given via a bottle.

Get Linked

Need advice about breastfeeding? Whether you are looking for information on getting started, a good breastfeeding class, or just information about how to breastfeed, pump, or otherwise manage, these links will guide you to the right spot.

FEEDING YOUR BABY

All of your feeding questions answered in one spot, from getting started to adding solids and more.

 http://about.com/pregnancy/feedingbaby

BREASTFEEDING CLASS

The materials for the handy breastfeeding class will arrive in your e-mail every week for six weeks. Here you will learn a variety of basic breastfeeding positions, tips and tricks. Also included are photos of breastfeeding positions and more.

 http://about.com/pregnancy/breastfeedingclass

WORKING AND NURSING

Need advice on breastfeeding and working? Here you'll find great information on pumping breast milk and storing it, particularly while working or traveling.

 http://about.com/pregnancy/workingnursing

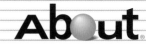

Chapter 13

Postpartum

The First Few Hours

Being handed your baby is such a magical moment. These first few moments are ones that you will not soon forget. The first few hours will quite likely be a blur. Planning ahead and knowing what to expect from your body and your baby can help you keep your wits about you and enjoy these exciting times.

Your body will do weird things. And that is the understatement of the year. With one last grand push, you are no longer a pregnant woman but a postpartum mother. The physical changes that go along with this transition are great.

For you, the immediate postpartum period will involve yet another exam of your bottom. You will be examined for bleeding, tearing, and any other problems that you may have experienced during birth. If you need any stitches, they will be done by your doctor or midwife at this time.

What happens with an epidural after you give birth?

▶ If you had an epidural, the catheter that was left in your back will be pulled out shortly after the birth, usually within an hour. How long it takes for you to regain the feeling in your legs and abdomen depends on things like how much medication you got and your reaction to it. This may take several hours. Most women tell me they start feeling some tingling first, then slowly regain the use of their legs. If you have any concerns about what you are feeling, do not hesitate to ask your anesthesiologist.

Vital signs, like your blood pressure, heart rate, and temperature will also be taken regularly for at least the first hour or so. Some of this will depend on where you gave birth and your practitioner's preferences. It will also depend on if you had any complications or medications, as these may affect your body in negative ways. If you do have problems, you will be monitored until all of the problems are resolved.

You may notice that your abdomen is no longer as large as it previously was. With the exit of your baby, the placenta, and the amniotic fluid, you have lost an incredible volume from your uterus, thus making it appear much smaller. The problem now? You probably still look six months pregnant and will for at least a few days. Your belly will also feel a bit like jelly.

After giving birth, chances are that you have a full bladder! Get up within the first hour to go to the bathroom, even if you don't feel like your bladder is full. You might be sore from positions you took in labor, but I also found it felt good to get up and move around, as so many other women do. Have someone like your doula or husband walk you to the bathroom in case you feel a bit shaky.

Recovering from cesarean surgery takes time. It is important to remember that a cesarean is surgery from which you need to recover, not simply another way to have a baby. Ensuring that you are taken care of physically provides you with more opportunities to be a mother to your new baby.

The first few hours after surgery will be spent in the recovery area, a postsurgery area where specially trained nurses will care for you and monitor you. Your baby, if he is healthy, should be allowed to remain in the recovery area with you.

Your IV line will usually stay in for at least twenty-four hours after surgery. This is used for fluids and medications as needed. Many hospitals will have you on a restricted diet for the first twelve to twenty-four hours following your surgery. Talk to your doctor about this if you are concerned.

You will likely spend at least four days in the hospital. During this time you will be monitored for normal postpartum issues, but also for surgical complications like infection or damage to other organs. This is done via checking vital signs, surgical wound checks, wound care, and blood work. If you are experiencing any pain or symptoms that are worrisome to you, be sure to ask for advice or help.

Pain management doesn't end at the birth. You are likely to feel sore, like you just exercised really hard for a very long time, because that is what you essentially did. You may have sore muscles you didn't know existed. (If you had surgery, with or without labor, you will also have a very sore abdomen and internal pain from the other incisions.)

Pain is not uncommon. If you are experiencing pain, consider what can be done to relieve it without medications that may make you drowsy. Try ice packs on your perineum to soothe this area. If pain medications are needed, ask for the least strong and smallest dose first and work your way up. Sometimes all you really need is an over-the-counter remedy.

One important concept is that of chasing pain, particularly after surgery. If you wait to take medications until you are in pain, then you will usually need to take more medication for a longer time. Try taking pain medication at the first sign of pain and then spend a day or two taking medication by the clock rather than by symptoms. This will help ensure adequate coverage of pain.

Bleeding after birth is normal. This is true no matter how your baby was born. The bleeding comes from the healing of the uterus at the site where your placenta was located. As your uterus begins the process of involution, or shrinking, you will bleed.

WHAT'S HOT

▶ After an abdominal surgery, like a cesarean section, I have found it helpful to splint the incision when moving, particularly when standing up. To do this, simply take a small pillow (which some hospitals supply) and brace your incision. While this will not remove all of the pain or fear when moving, it can drastically reduce them. I found it helped me to not feel like my intestines were going to fall out.

This blood is called lochia. Your lochia starts off being bright red and heavier than a period at first, usually with blood clots, for the first day or so. This usually slows after the first few days. You will notice the color generally becoming pink or clear. It will last up to six weeks postpartum.

Some women notice that their bleeding gets heavier or darker when they are physically active. This is generally a sign that you need to take it easy. Slowing back down for a day or two will usually see the lochia going back to the lighter color.

You should never use tampons in the early postpartum period. Generally we say you can use tampons again at your first period after your baby, which may be some time away. You should use sanitary napkins. Change them frequently to stay clean and dry.

Your baby's first hours are important. This is not only a time to greet your newborn and get to know her, but a time of great physical change in her body as she learns to survive and thrive in the world outside of her mother.

The American Academy of Pediatrics (AAP) recommends that you begin breastfeeding in the first thirty minutes of your baby's life. This provides your baby with the skin-to-skin warmth she needs. It provides you with an up-close and personal meeting with your new baby.

If you had a home birth, you've got more say in what happens. You will be able to move around more freely after birth. At some point after you have given birth, your midwife will do a very through newborn examination. This will include a look at every extremity, measuring and weighing, any injections or medications needed by your baby, checking out her eyes, heart, ears, genitals, and everything else. Be sure to watch and ask questions about what is being done and why. My midwife gave me a copy of this exam sheet to take with me to my baby's first pediatrician appointment the next day.

Your midwife will generally stay for at least a few hours to monitor you and your baby. They will give you instructions on how and when to call them should you need them, though generally they will return the next day to check on you and baby.

The First Few Days

The first few days after the birth are interesting. You're experiencing so much physically and emotionally. It can feel very overwhelming. It can leave you wondering what is normal and what isn't normal.

Be sure to call your practitioner if you experience any of the following problems:

- Fever
- Heavy bleeding (more than a pad every half hour)
- Foul-smelling discharge
- Problems urinating
- Bleeding from your incision
- Your cesarean incision becomes red and more painful
- Breastfeeding problems or pain
- Feeling dizzy or passing out
- Feeling out of breath
- Swelling or tenderness in your legs
- Any other concerns you have

During the first few days after birth, you should focus on your baby, you, your family, and other basics. You will need to eat and sleep. You should take care of your body to help it heal. Every day you will begin to feel stronger and more confident in your parenting and in general.

▶ Keeping your baby warm is an important task in the first few hours. The easiest place to warm your baby is skin-to-skin with you. You can simply snuggle baby at your breast under your shirt or gown. If you need to, you can add extra warmth by covering both of you with a thin blanket. If you aren't feeling well or need to go to the bathroom, you can also have your husband hold the baby skin-to-skin.

It is normal to feel overwhelmed and concerned about doing it all. Do not let this keep you down. You are not expected to do everything or be the perfect mother or wife. Simply do what you need to do to get by during the first days.

If your partner is able to take some time off from work, that can be very helpful for everyone. This means that you can have some help at night and during the day. He can feel more connected to the family and help establish a routine for your lives.

A postpartum doula is someone who can really be of help to your family. A postpartum doula will generally spend a few hours a few days a week getting your house in order and helping with light housework and meals. It can be a huge relief to know that dinner will be served and everyone has clean clothes, particularly if you don't have to do it.

Physical issues are prevalent in the first few days. Within the first few days after giving birth, you will probably have your first bowel movement. This scares many women because they are worried about pain and injury with the first bowel movement. My advice is to eat lots of fruits and veggies to make for a softer stool. You can usually do this with diet and water and not medications. Some practitioners do routinely recommend or prescribe stool softeners to new moms.

When the time comes, just relax and let the stool pass slowly. Don't be concerned with injuring any sutures you may have in your perineum. If you see blood with your stool, it is most likely from hemorrhoids or your lochia. This will generally get better as time goes on.

Your baby will adjust in the first few days. He will show you all of his reflexes and begin to interact with you. You can watch him stare at you and see him follow your voice. These first few days are precious and fun, but also a time of great adjustment.

You might not be used to round the-clock parenting yet. So the change from simply getting up to go to the bathroom and go back to bed at the end of pregnancy is very different from the feed me, change me, love me routine that the first days bring.

If during birth or right after birth your baby had a large bowel movement, she may not need to have another for a while. After the first few days, the number of stools your baby has a day can vary greatly. Though usually a baby at this age will have at least one stool a day.

The First Few Weeks

The first few weeks after birth are hectic to say the least. While it seems like there is a lot of physical downtime, the mental and emotional work is great. During this period of time you are working to incorporate a new being into your life, whether it's baby number one or baby number five. You are also processing the birth experience, which will take time to really grasp.

The sleep deprivation can drive you crazy. The old adage about sleeping when the baby sleeps is so true. Yet it is often difficult to lie down and take a nap in the middle of the day. Even if you can't sleep, I'd urge you to try, even if you only rest for short periods with or without sleep. This will help you regenerate and have the strength for activity in the middle of the night.

During the day you might find that you sleep better at a certain time, like maybe you sleep best by sleeping in until a later time. Have your husband get up alone or with other children, even if you usually join him or help them. This will allow you to sleep more hours. Find something flexible and real that works for your family.

TOOLS YOU NEED

▶ Sometimes after birth you may find that you are suffering from negative thoughts about the experience of birth. Perhaps you feel you were treated disrespectfully or that your wishes were not heard or acted upon. *Rebounding from Childbirth*, by Lynn Madsen, is a great resource for you if you are dealing with a negative birth experience. My take-home message was that it is okay to be happy that you have a healthy baby and disappointed with the journey that got you there.

There are no magic cures for the sleep issues that surround new motherhood. Remember that your baby is not waking up to be spiteful, but rather because of real needs. Trust your instincts and do what feels right by way of your baby. Don't be tempted to listen to others who want to tell you that they have the perfect answer if you do everything their way, particularly if that is against your beliefs.

Crying babies are loud.   Even when yours is just whimpering, you may find that you are very tuned in. Babies cry for lots of reasons, including these:

- Hungry
- Wet/dirty
- Cold/hot
- Overstimulated
- Lonely
- Tired
- Hurt

Crying and sleep do not have to go together. New babies need a lot of sleep, but what most books don't tell you is that the large number of hours that they sleep are usually in small spurts, not long marathons. Many people will try to tell you that allowing your baby to cry for hours on end and to ignore the feelings you have to comfort your child is the only way to teach your baby to sleep. Remember that babies have many needs throughout the day and night that aren't always convenient or able to be timed. If your baby is crying, you need to respond to her. Sleep experts who used to believe that "crying it out" was appropriate have now reversed themselves and said that you should follow your gut and heart and respond to your baby's cries.

TOOLS YOU NEED

▶ New babies aren't meant to cry for hours on end. There are many sleep "methods" that involve crying babies, though recently experts have said maybe they were wrong to advise parents to allow their babies to cry so much. It always hurt me as a mother to hear my baby cry; my mothering instinct said it was wrong. I found some great advice in Elizabeth Pantley's *No Cry Sleep Solution* for helping make nighttime easier on everyone.

Getting out is important. I personally recommend getting out of the house, even for a small trip, pretty soon after having your baby. My husband and I like to go out to eat with the baby in a sling. We usually do this the first week after the baby is born.

Lunch winds up being a good time to go because most places aren't crowded and you are not tired from your day. Getting out of the house helps lift your spirits in many ways. It also helps if you take a short trip to see how mobile babies really are, even in the beginning.

When going out with your baby, remember to go easy on yourself. Plan short trips at first. Always leave lots of extra time for diaper changes, feeding, and just plain time to do everything that goes along with bringing baby out, like putting on a sling, removing baby from her car seat, or unfolding the stroller.

Yes, there is sex postpartum. Stressing out about the when and the how will only drive you crazy. So try as best you can to just let it happen naturally.

Before you have sex, you need to be sure that your uterus and perineum have healed. Generally speaking you should no longer be bleeding or have staples or sutures present. This goes for vaginal or cesarean birth. For many women this will be around six weeks postpartum.

You might obviously feel a bit nervous about having sex for the first time after having your baby. Remember to talk to your partner about it. Being able to take the time to talk about your nerves and his are important. The keys to a successful and pleasant first post-birth encounter involve time, patience, and respect. Be vocal about what feels good as well as what doesn't feel good.

If you're overly anxious, try easing back into a physical relationship. Holding hands while you watch television or playing footsie

TOOLS YOU NEED

▸ Keep your diaper bag stocked and ready to grab as you walk out the door. You might find that you are more willing to go places spur of the moment than you thought, even if it's a quick trip to the grocery or pediatrician. Knowing all you have to do is grab your well-stocked diaper bag and put your new baby in the car seat and you're ready can mentally ease your mind about the transition. It also helps you get out of the house, which can do wonders for your mental health.

while you eat dinner are great ways to physically reconnect without being too physical or sexual.

Many new mothers complain about feeling "touched out." This can be very real. Figure out how to differentiate the touches or find a time when you are more open to be touched. Remember all touches are not alike.

If you take the time to have an orgasm before intercourse, then you will be more lubricated. If lubrication is a concern of yours, you are allowed to use water-soluble lubricants like KY Jelly. This is something that will help lubricate your vagina and will not interfere with any birth control method you might be using using.

Before having sex, remember to bring along your sense of humor. Babies seem to wake up just as you're getting amorous with your honey. My husband would try to tend to our little one while I simply did nothing. Having nothing to do helped me to stay relaxed and just lay around for a bit. This always made me more likely to be interested once the baby was settled.

You've got one last trip to your practitioner.   After nine long months, it can be very hard to say goodbye to your doctor or midwife. But after about six weeks you'll be seeing him or her for the last time, at least until your annual exam.

Your postpartum visit will seem more like your annual exam, except that you have a cute baby to bring with you. You will have your pap smear and your breast exam. Your midwife or doctor will also want to check on your healing process from birth, either vaginally or by cesarean.

In addition to the physical exam, you will have an opportunity to talk about the birth of your baby. Maybe you've had some questions come up now that you've had time to think about what happened. This is a nice, neutral time to ask these questions and to get answers.

You will want to be sure to discuss the following with your practitioner:

- Breastfeeding
- Postpartum birth control
- Resuming sexual relations
- Exercise and weight loss
- Postpartum lab work that may be needed
- Unresolved questions about your birth
- When you should be seen again

Postpartum Emotions

With the roller coaster of emotions that is pregnancy, you would hope that postpartum would be a bit more calm. Unfortunately there are many emotions that go along with being a new mom. Joy. Excitement. Sadness. Fear. The majority of mothers will experience some emotional unrest in the first weeks after giving birth.

The baby blues start a few days after birth. About 80 percent of mothers will experience this mild form of depression, which normally goes away after a few weeks without treatment. The baby blues are mostly hormonal and physical in nature. You'll know you've got the baby blues if you do the following:

- Cry for no reason
- Have mood swings
- Feel clingy or dependent
- Feel sad
- Have an inability to concentrate

While the baby blues happen to a large percentage of new mothers, it doesn't make it feel any better. If you find you have

BEFORE YOUR APPOINTMENT

▶ Discuss with your partner what type of birth control you are interested in with the birth of your baby. Perhaps your old method worked fine and you intend to go back to that one. Or if you're in the market for a different method, bring your partner with you to your six-week checkup to discuss new options.

the baby blues, try to say something to someone. A good childbirth class will go over the signs of baby blues and other postpartum issues so that your husband or others can spot it and help you too.

Since medical treatment isn't necessary, you may wonder what someone can do to help you. Having someone to help with the house, fix meals, and do general day-to-day household business can be helpful. Sometimes it's nice to take a long hot shower and rest to help rebuild your strength and buffer you from some sleepless nights. Remembering to ask for help can be the hardest part of postpartum, but the baby blues will quickly bring you to your knees if you don't get some physical help from others.

Postpartum depression is more than the baby blues. Luckily it doesn't happen to everyone. Only about 15 to 20 percent of mothers get postpartum depression. It differs from the baby blues in that it can occur gradually anytime over the first year after giving birth. Because of this, it may seem very subtle. The following are a few potential signs of postpartum depression:

- ○ Lack of concentration
- ○ Excessive worry
- ○ Anxiety
- ○ Short temper
- ○ Excessive fatigue
- ○ Feelings of being overwhelmed
- ○ Decreased sexual interest/libido
- ○ Weight loss or gain
- ○ Lack of feeling or awkwardness around baby
- ○ Hopelessness

Postpartum depression is treatable. It may involve counseling, medication, lifestyle changes or a combination of all three. But there is life after postpartum depression.

An experience with postpartum depression may leave you fearful about having another child. Be sure to talk to your practitioner about planning another baby. While you are at a higher risk of having postpartum depression, there are things you can do to make your next postpartum experience very different.

Personally, I found that by ensuring I had a lot of help postpartum, by way of my husband having a couple of weeks off and hiring a postpartum doula, I was able to avoid another nasty bout with postpartum depression. My midwife stayed in close contact with us, and my husband was reminded of what to look for to help be her eyes and ears when she wasn't around. I had some rough days, but nothing like the months and months of depression I had the first time. So get help, educate those around you, and don't isolate yourself.

Living Life with Baby

Having a baby changes everything about your life. You probably knew that. Several people probably told you that. But the actual experience is usually different than what you thought it would be.

Eventually you will find a new routine for your life. You will find that you learn a lot about yourself as a mother. Learning to trust your mothering instincts and read your baby will give you a sense of accomplishment. It takes time. Don't be stressed out over not feeling settled into motherhood at a week or a month. Generally speaking, it will take you a year to feel your new sense of normal, though your life drastically calms at around six months postpartum.

Learn to take your baby with you places. Learning how to sling and carry your baby can help you feel more confident in being out

ELSEWHERE ON THE WEB

▶ Postpartum Support International (PSI) (on the Web at www.postpartum.net) is a great resource for new families. Their site offers great articles on various aspects of postpartum mood disorders, including a special section just for fathers. Here you can also find out how to find local help.

in public. Your baby will also feel more secure close to you or Dad when in a new environment.

Venture out alone occasionally. I used to love to go grocery shopping. I know that sounds weird, particularly if you know how I hate to cook. But my sister and I would go to an all-night megastore at 11 P.M. and walk and talk through every aisle for a couple of hours. It was a great time for us to get out alone while accomplishing something that needed to be done.

Playing with your baby is important. Even before your baby can talk or walk, she will interact with you. You need to take the lead on this and engage her when possible. The good news is that this not a difficult or complex task.

Talking to your baby throughout the day is a great form of stimulation for her brain. Talking may come naturally, or it may not. An easy way to start up a one-sided conversation with your baby is to simply explain what you are doing. This easy dialogue of daily activities will help you feel more at ease with conversing and help you know what to say when you're at a loss for words. Don't stress, the rest will come.

Read and sing to your baby on a regular basis as well. This can be the beginning of a lifelong love of reading, but more importantly it is a nice way to bond with your baby. Consider having Dad read a short story before bedtime as you begin to have a bedtime routine. This bedtime reading can last for years.

As your baby grows, there are other ways that you will learn to play and communicate with your baby. We enjoyed doing baby sign language with our last five kids. It was fun and easy and helped them communicate their thoughts before their bodies would allow them to speak. We still use it today to communicate in large crowds—signing the word "no" is a lot less interruptive than screaming it and it is just as effective.

No matter how you play or communicate with your baby, take the time to enjoy it. Everyone tells you that kids are only young once or that they grow up really quickly—that is because it is the truth. One day you'll blink and realize that your tiny, helpless newborn is sitting up or walking.

Finding your new normal takes time. Think of it this way. Having a baby is not being about your world changing completely; it's about accepting the baby into your lives and helping him be a part of your world. This is much easier to do than to drastically change everything.

New babies need so very little. They need food, diapers, and love. It can be easy to fall into the trap of worrying about all the equipment to contain your baby, but remember that it is much easier to incorporate the baby into your life if you carry the baby in a sling or other carrier. This is partially because there's less stuff to haul around, but it's more because you are there to respond to your child's needs.

Try not to think of having a new baby as your previous life ending and a new life beginning. It is really more of an extension of your current life. Your life becomes richer and more full with the addition of your baby. Your relationships and world will change, but become a more cohesive unit when you keep this philosophy and your baby close to your heart.

TOOLS YOU NEED

▶ **One of the hardest things to fathom about the early postpartum period is how many different emotions you can have and how quickly your moods can change.** A book that I love, as do my readers, is *Laughter and Tears: The Emotional Life of a New Mother,* by Elisabeth Bing and Libby Coleman, Ph.D. This warm and thoughtful book talks about everything that can go through your mind as a new mom, and it includes letters from other new moms. It's an easy book to have by the bed and to read a bit out of as a pick-me-up. I've also found it helpful for dads and others dealing with a new baby in their lives.

Get Linked

Newborns are hard work and lots of fun all rolled into one adorable package. There is a lot to learn about your baby and how to care for him. I've gathered up some information on taking care of you, your baby, and your family below, including a handy e-mail course for new babies.

NEWBORN BABIES

Newborn babies need everything from you. From diaper changes to baths and beyond, your baby has needs that you need to meet. I've got help for you. You'll find charts on caring for baby's umbilical cord, to baby-care basics like bathing, holding, and feeding.

 http://about.com/pregnancy/newborns

PHYSICAL RECOVERY AFTER BIRTH

To answer all of your tough questions about getting back to normal after having a baby, including your immediate physical recovery from either a vaginal birth or a cesarean, physical exercise, and more.

 http://about.com/pregnancy/recovery

POSTPARTUM DEPRESSION

Postpartum depression (PPD) is real. Here you'll find a screening tool to help you see if you need to seek help as well as resources and the basics of postpartum depression and beyond.

 http://about.com/pregnancy/postpartumdepress

Chapter 14

Dad's Role and Other Support

Helping Dad Survive Pregnancy

While you were undoubtedly surprised to find out you were pregnant, Dad-to-be was probably even more shocked by the news. I've found even when my husband and I were planning a pregnancy he was always the most shocked about the pregnancy.

Settling into the pregnancy takes time for everyone. Once the initial shock is over you may find that Dad doesn't think about pregnancy as much as you do. This is partially because it isn't happening to his body. And other than listening to you talk about being pregnant, he isn't reminded of it on a daily basis.

She's pregnant. We're pregnant. Not sure which to say? It probably depends on whom you are asking. Many women tell me they feel all warm and fuzzy that their man wants to share in

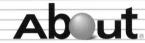

▶ Dad may find himself gaining weight and bloating just like you. Perhaps he's even been known to have morning sickness and cravings. This is known as Couvade syndrome. It is a sympathetic pregnancy experienced by the father. Supposedly this means he's very emotionally connected, and the good news is that it does go away after birth.

the experience, even to the point of claiming he is pregnant, too. However, it's probably not the right time to make this claim if you're not the one throwing up.

Dad's involvement in the pregnancy involves more than just how you phrase it. He needs to actively do what he can to take part in the pregnancy. This can involve various things from helping you when you aren't feeling well to showing an interest in the pregnancy.

Dads should read about pregnancy. Suggest that he find a couple of sources to read about the changes that happen to both of you in pregnancy. He might even surprise you and read sources you don't read. He might casually drop into the conversation one day something amazing about how the baby is growing or doing that week. This will really strengthen the bond between you.

There are books out there specifically written for dads. Try a couple of those on for size. If books are not his thing, there are Web sites galore. Some have weekly e-mails that he can subscribe to or classes he can take online.

Reading and learning about pregnancy helps him form his own opinions. He can participate in discussions and not have to ask you every five seconds what you are talking about. He'll know and be able to help with the decision-making process.

Don't be concerned about dependence issues. Sometimes mothers-to-be feel a bit more connected during pregnancy. In trying to facilitate that bond with your partner, they might sense that you are a bit more needy or clingy. If you have been independent up until this point, don't fear. You are not making a sweeping change; instead, you just trying to gather extra support as you sort through everything going on in your mind and your body. Feeling that extra bit of support by sticking close to your partner is a positive thing for both of you.

Concerns Dads Have About Pregnancy

Pregnancy can be such a swiftly changing time. From the mood swings to the rapidly expanding abdomen, everything seems to happen so quickly. There's barely time for him to worry about one thing before another thing comes up. The basic fact is that worry in pregnancy is normal for anyone.

Sex is a huge concern of dads-to-be. He will likely have many questions about sex in pregnancy, with the safety of his wife and the baby being the highest level of concern. The good news is that except for very special circumstances like premature labor and other severe problems in labor, all types of sexual activities are completely acceptable.

The good news about pregnant sex is that there is no birth control to worry about. While technically you were not using birth control when you were trying to get pregnant, you still had a task to perform. Now you can make love and not worry about birth control, ovulation, or anything else.

With the added vaginal lubrication of pregnancy, many dads say that sex is very pleasurable for them. Since you are able to have orgasms more easily, you may become multiorgasmic for the first time. Dads write to say they really enjoy this aspect of pregnant sex because it makes them feel really good that she's having such a good time.

Most sexual positions and acts are perfectly safe in pregnancy. This includes oral sex. Some women feel uncomfortable with oral sex in pregnancy because of the increased vaginal discharge. You can also incorporate a shower into your lovemaking sessions to help decrease the amount of extra discharge.

ASK YOUR GUIDE

When should we start thinking about paternity leave?

▶ Think about paternity leave early. Does his company have a policy? What about the state in which you live? Have you considered the Family and Medical Leave Act (FMLA)? Knowing what your rights are and what you have available will help you plan for the birth. It will also help his employer if he has his ongoing projects ready to be handed over. Most dads who didn't take time off in the beginning say they regret that, not to mention what the moms say.

▶ **If he wants to learn more about pregnancy, he should try attending all the prenatal appointments that he can. Then he also has an opportunity to ask questions of your midwife or doctor and learn from them. He will also be able to ask his own questions and get the joy of watching his baby grow. If he can't make every visit, make as many as he can, perhaps hit at least one per trimester and big appointments like ultrasounds or testing.**

If your nipples are very sensitive, you may want to avoid having him touch them, even accidentally. If you normally want him to touch them, be sure he asks first. If your nipples wind up being very sensitive, sometimes wearing a thin cotton jog bra can help make them less sensitive.

Look and listen for the emotional and physical changes in pregnancy. There are many, but they do not have to stop your love life. Simply figuring out how to work around everything and doing what you can works for most couples.

As each trimester brings new changes, you will have to adapt. Figuring out what you both need is usually accomplished with ease by discussing what you're thinking. The biggest thing is to keep communicating.

Many dads worry about being good fathers. So if he is worried about what kind of dad he will be, he is not alone. Take the fact that he cares whether or not that he is a good father as a positive sign. Now what can he do about it?

Reading books on parenting and attending classes aimed at helping dads with some of the basics are a good step. If he has any friends with kids, particularly small babies, perhaps he can come play with the baby to get a handle on some of the smaller tasks like diaper changes.

These are all helpful things to physically prepare for the tasks of raising your baby. But sometimes the best preparation is an emotional one. Ask yourself some questions about how you were parented, what you liked, what you would do differently. Think of ways to talk about this together. Maybe have him ask himself the same questions and sit down with your answers for discussions.

Can you afford a baby? You may be longing for a suite of baby furniture that costs an arm and a leg. He's now thinking about food and shelter. But you know that down the road is camp and college. How will you make it?

Remember babies do not really cost that much money. You do not need every latest and greatest thing out there for babies. You really can do with just some minor purchases, most of which do not even need to be new to work.

Hopefully prior to pregnancy you checked your health insurance to make sure that maternity coverage was included in your health policy. This should cover the majority of your health needs during the pregnancy. You will be expected to pay any deductibles or copayments as defined by your insurance.

Your doctor or midwife generally provides one bill for all of your pregnancy, birth, and postpartum care. You will probably need a copayment for these services as a bundle, rather than a copayment per visit. Lab work or blood work done someplace other than your practitioner's office may be an additional copay. This goes for any prenatal testing done outside of that bundle of pregnancy care.

Ultrasounds may or may not be covered by your insurance. This will depend on the reason for the ultrasound. If it is to provide you medical care, like diagnosing a suspected ectopic pregnancy or finding a cause of bleeding, it will most likely be covered but subject to a copayment. If it is a routine screening with no medical reason behind it, then you may be stuck with that bill or choose not to have the test. Check with your insurance to see what it covers.

Your hospital or birth center bill will most likely be a separate fee, thus requiring an additional copayment. Many insurance plans will have you pay 20 percent of the hospital fees up to a certain point rather than a copayment. Talk to the hospital or birth center about the fees and what you will need to pay up front. Make a payment arrangement as soon as possible to avoid larger bills. Be

ELSEWHERE ON THE WEB

▶ Financial calculators are fun ways to calculate expected expenses, making sure you have enough insurance coverage or calculating a due date. I'd highly recommend playing around with some of those calculators, like those on the Kiplinger's Web site (www.kiplinger .com). It can provide you with a world of information on your financial status.

sure to ask what services you are paying for in that prepaid bill. Things that you may need covered are the following:

- Labor and birth room and staff
- Hospital supplies (disposable items, medications, monitoring devices)
- Operating room for cesarean
- Assistant surgeon for cesarean
- Neonatologist for cesarean or complicated birth
- Anesthesia, cesarean or vaginal birth (if needed)
- Lab work before, during, and after birth
- Newborn nursery care, even if your baby stays with you
- Postpartum room and staff
- Any special tests for mom and/or baby
- Specialized nursery care

A hospital birth costs about $8,000 for an uncomplicated vaginal birth. That number is considerably higher for a cesarean birth because of the surgery and added surgeons, medications, and the operating room. You must also stay several additional days to heal after the cesarean birth.

Birth centers tend to cost less. This is because there are fewer interventions used and shorter postpartum stays. They also bundle services into one fee many times. Be sure to ask what your fees cover. Insurance companies often cover birth center births, so do check with your insurance company.

If you are planning a home birth, the payment for the services of the midwife normally cover nearly everything that you will need to pay. You may be asked to pay $50 to $80 for a birth kit, which includes all of the sterile supplies used by the midwife, like gloves, cord clamps, and pads. There may be cases in which you need to pay a fee for the assistant midwife as well. This varies greatly.

Usually a home birth is several thousand dollars less than a hospital birth. One mom wrote me to say she was prepared to pay out of pocket for her home birth. Luckily she found out she didn't have to do that because her insurance company was going to pick up most of the cost of her care. I'd recommend calling and writing your insurance company. When faced with the decision of whether or not to pay for a very expensive hospital birth or your lower-cost home birth, many make exceptions to policies to pay. If not, ask your midwife about payment plans.

New babies also are fairly inexpensive. Breastfeeding can help you save even more money. This goes way beyond the savings from buying your baby food. Because breastfed babies are healthier, they have fewer doctor visits and fewer medications. This also translates into your taking off less time to watch a sick baby or to go to the pediatrician.

Support During Birth

Gone are the days when most dads spend the hours of labor and birth in the waiting room. Now the waiting rooms are filled with extended family. Dads are right in the trenches with mom.

He should be prepared to help you in labor. Talk to him about what your expectations are for him in labor. Then tell him what your preferences are for labor. See where you can meet in the middle.

For example, you may expect that he will remind you to go the bathroom, change position, figure out which position you should be in, run interference with the nursing staff, rub your back, and a whole host of other responsibilities. He may have been thinking he'd be responsible for driving you to the hospital or birth center and nothing else. You need to work together on this topic.

ASK YOUR GUIDE

All I seem to think about is pregnancy. Is this normal?

▶ You probably do not think of much else these days. Everything is filtered through your pregnancy brain. The experience that you are having and the experience that he is having are very different at this point. Even later in pregnancy, when the physical changes are very evident in your body, he is still not dealing with it the same way. Be sure to let him know that you'd like to talk about something else occasionally by trying to shut off the pregnancy part of your brain for a few minutes.

A dad wrote me to ask why his wife was suggesting a doula. He felt like a doula wasn't needed. But when he heard everything that his wife expected, he relented. He just wrote to say that his experience with the doula was wonderful and that all babies born in his family would have doula care. Their doula took over all the tasks he didn't want to do, but also was able to provide him with gentle guidance to help him participate fully and have his wife feel supported by him.

Worried about the blood and body fluids? Birth can be bloody and involve other fluids. If he is squeamish, you may be concerned about his catching sight of blood, body fluids, or the rest of the potential medical stuff.

Try not to be overly concerned about the sight of blood in birth. Generally there is only a bit of blood and usually not until the very end, after the birth of the baby. By then he will be so entranced with his wife and new child, he won't even notice. I do advise that he should avoid looking at the placenta if he is a bit nervous about blood.

What about medications in labor? No, he can't have any! If you have decided that you do not want to have medications in labor, then you will be using other forms of assistance, usually in the form of comfort measures. It will be up to Dad and your doula, if you have one, to help keep you as comfortable as possible during labor.

It is not his place to jump in and tell you that you must have medications or procedures you don't want. And labor is not the time to have this discussion. This should be talked about well in advance of labor. If he knows that he is not going to be able to provide you the support you need, be sure you have someone else available to help you. In the same vein, he should not be able to tell you that you should not have medications.

Attending a childbirth class together will help you deal with many of these issues. In class, you will most likely do some birth planning and values clarification exercises to help the two of you talk openly about what you are expecting from the birth experience both in terms of the overall outcome and in terms of support from one another.

Once the baby is born, she will go to your abdomen. Here you can both look at her and touch her. If the cord is long enough, the baby can go directly to the breast. Cover the baby with a dry towel and keep her skin-to-skin with you to help her stay warm. This allows the baby to have access to nurse and is the best place to warm her.

The hospital staff may be interested in doing their bit to put on hospital ID bracelets, administer eye drops, or injections as required by your state. They may also wish to weigh and measure your baby. Only you and your husband can decide when you are ready to have this done, and with the exception of medical emergencies, there is no reason it can't be done while the baby is with you.

Feel free to take pictures and celebrate! Remember to ask someone to take your picture as a threesome. The flood of emotions he will feel is amazing. He's just been there as his baby is born. He got to help his wife in labor. And now he's a dad.

Some dads are concerned about watching the birth. I've heard this from dads on the Internet as well as in my doula practice. This common concern is one that needs to be discussed with your partner.

Is his concern about watching you in pain? Is it about seeing the baby born? Or even being in the room? One of the easiest compromises, if seeing the birth is your concern, or his, is to have him be in the room, but up near your head so that he does not

TOOLS YOU NEED

▶ *The Birth Partner,* by Penny Simkin, was written with dads and other labor support people in mind. It is a handy guide to the last weeks of pregnancy, with a particular emphasis on the labor and birth. I love the handy pages that are marked as quick reference sheets. You can easily flip to these pages and get fast facts on dealing with nearly any situation in labor or birth. This will be an easy way to help your partner build his confidence in supporting you as you give birth. Be sure to read it early and pack it in your birth bag.

have to look as the baby is coming out. This prevents him from seeing the birth but makes him available to support you in labor and to be one of the first people to greet your new baby. Many dads find this to be the best compromise for the birth situation.

If it is determined that a cesarean birth is the way your baby needs to be born, he will most likely be allowed into the operating room. He will only not be allowed into the room if it is an emergency surgery, if you have general anesthesia (go to sleep), or if you do not want him there.

Normally Dad will be given a set of scrubs or a paper suit to wear to cover his clothes. He will also be given a mask for his face. Booties and a hair covering will also be worn into the operating suite. Be sure to let him know to ask for help in putting these on if he is unsure of how they go on. Typically these will be given to him while they take you to the operating room and he will wait outside until they come to get him.

If he finds himself sitting behind a curtain for a cesarean and the anesthesiologist tells him to stand up so he can see your baby be born, he shouldn't panic. You really can't see much except the baby being born at this point. But he also doesn't have to make the choice to stand up.

Once your baby is born, she will usually be quickly taken to the warmer. Typically this warmer is either inside the operating room or just outside the operating room. Here she will be dried off and helped to start breathing. This can range from brisk rubbing of her skin and oxygen to more intensive medical assistance such as intubation, where the staff will breathe for her. Dad is allowed to go to the warmer to watch, take pictures, and hold the baby. Be sure to have Dad bring her to you as soon as she is ready.

Once there, be sure to turn her face toward yours with Dad's help, and pull any thick blankets away from her face so that you can see. It is very difficult to see while you are lying down on your back, so he may have to hold the baby at different angles to help you see.

Once you are in the recovery room, he can help you start to breastfeed. It is best if you unwrap your baby and place her skin-to-skin next to you. Be sure you are both covered with a dry blanket. You should probably keep the baby's hat on as well. Your husband will need to support your arms by using more pillows to keep the baby in place. (See Chapter 12 for more information on first feedings.)

Managing Postpartum

You have probably been told that postpartum is no fun. That is really an unfair characterization of these early first days of your new baby's life. The truth of the matter is that if you plan well and know what to expect, this can be the best time of your life.

Sleep with a new baby is possible.   One of your biggest fears about having a new baby may be the lack of sleep that is likely to follow. This is particularly common in dads-to-be. I'm here to tell you that it is an important concern for a very real potential problem.

While everyone may tell you to sleep when the baby sleeps, that is very hard to actually do. Babies simply don't sleep like grown-ups do. It can be easier to get that daytime nap in if you and your family feel that other needs like food and laundry are taken care of before nap time. Your choices are either to ignore those feelings or to be sure these are addressed early in the day.

Having meals prepared ahead of time can be a blessing for these days. You can also learn what meals are easily thrown in the slow cooker. Or delegate the responsibility of dinner to a friend, family member, or your postpartum doula.

My idea of tackling laundry and my husband's are vastly different. I don't feel like you can put a load in unless you intend to see

ASK YOUR GUIDE

Does lighting affect a baby's sleep?

▶ Yes. I personally advise turning on as few lights as possible. A small night light near where you will feed the baby is usually fine once breastfeeding is established. Also model for your baby that this is night time and not play time. You can do this by keeping a soft voice and limiting stimulating contact like rattles, toys, bright lights, and things of that nature.

it through to completion before doing anything else. This means I'd have to stay awake. My husband taught me that it's perfectly fine to throw a load in as soon as you get up, and then ignore it until later morning or afternoon when you can throw it in the dryer. If we're talking basic clothes here, there is also no reason to immediately rescue them from the dryer—they can wait.

Nighttime sleeping is a completely different ball of wax. Studies show that parents who sleep the closest to their babies get the most sleep, particularly in the early months. That means if your baby is in her own crib in a separate room down the hall, you are likely to get less sleep than if she is in your room, either in your bed or in a bassinet near your bed.

Having your baby close at hand helps you hear those early cues for feeding. Remember, crying is a late sign of hunger. By the time the baby is crying, you will have to work twice as hard to calm, feed, change, and calm her again for bed before she will get back to sleep. By being able to rouse at earlier cues, you can quickly and easily feed the baby.

Baby care is for everyone. This means that Dad can help diaper and bathe your baby. In fact, other than physically breastfeeding, he can do a lot of the baby care himself or in conjunction with you. Lots of dads tell me that bath time is their favorite part of baby care.

He can also help by doing baby's laundry. Be sure to tell him if there is a special detergent being used for your baby's items. Other than using a special detergent, the only other thing our family does is to do the rinse cycle twice. This goes for cloth diapers as well as clothes.

Carrying the baby is a great way to bond. I love to see a daddy carrying a baby—it's so sweet. Most dads will also tell you that carrying their baby is a great way to not only bond with the baby but to reconnect after a long day at work or being away.

There are many types of carriers that can be used for carrying your baby. Some are more like slings or pouches, while others are backpacks. The type of carrier you use will depend on the age of your baby and how well he can hold up his head. Be sure to select an appropriate carrier based on these factors. Most moms and dads actually share carriers, so finding one that accommodates your body and his is preferred if this is what you will be doing. Slings are best suited for this sharing, in my opinion. They are also the most versatile.

Here is a checklist of things you and your husband should know how to do for your baby:

- Diaper the baby
- Do laundry for the baby
- Install the car seat and/or base
- Properly place baby in the car seat
- Contact the pediatrician
- Put a breast pump together
- Warm breast milk
- Prepare bottles
- Burp the baby
- Swaddle baby
- "Wear" the baby
- Fold and unfold the stroller

ELSEWHERE ON THE WEB

▶ Is Dad-to-be in need of some good fatherly advice or role model? Look no further than the Ask Dr. Sears Web site with all its information on fathering, at www.askdrsears .com. I love the handy information from other dads to help put your mind and his at ease about issues you are not likely to see elsewhere, like nurturing your baby as a father.

The Family's Support System

You've heard the quote about it taking a village to raise a child. Well, it couldn't be more true. A new family needs so much support, even if this baby is not your first. You will need need all kinds of support, including physical, emotional, and mental. The good news is that finding this support does not have to be difficult. Still, proper planning is very important. Be sure to ask for help early and often.

Grandparents are often great sources of help. If they are close and physically able, you can use grandparents for all kinds of assistance. They are often willing to come over with a meal and help with household chores. They are also particularly good at helping with older children.

If the grandparents aren't particularly helpful because they want to come over and hold the baby while you do the housework, you probably want to have a talk with them about what would be most helpful. If they can't offer you the kind of support you need, invite them over for social visits as you are able and find help elsewhere.

Other family members might be available. They may also be closer to your age, like your siblings. This may mean they have current information and recent practice. Advice of this nature can be invaluable at a time when your life is a bit upside down.

Be sure to ask them about what works for them and what doesn't. They might have great advice on buying baby products or even have some available for loan. Ask them where they get baby care services like a lactation consultant, pediatrician, or day care.

Once your baby is born, be sure to turn to these family members for physical help as well. Can they cook a meal? Do some laundry? Are they available to help with older siblings while you're having the baby? This also works great for play dates after baby as well.

Friends are often like extended family. The good news about friends is that they are probably like-minded and easier to talk to in some ways than even your family. The help they can provide is much like other family members with meals and the scoop on having a baby, assuming they have one or more themselves.

We tend to not want to impose on our friends. Remember, friendship is a give and take. What you allow them to do for you today is what you are able to repay them at a later date. Don't hesitate to ask for help with small errands like quick trips to the grocery store or to the post office. Ask for meals. And even ask for company at home!

Professionals are also available for help. For example, you might hire a maid to help with housekeeping chores. You might find a babysitter to ease the burden of the late afternoon with the older siblings. And a diaper service is a great idea to have clean diapers delivered right to your door.

Your parents might regale you with stories of baby nurses, though there are relatively few of these left. What has replaced the baby nurse is called a postpartum doula. This is someone, usually a woman, trained to assist new families as they welcome a baby.

The duties of a postpartum doula include light housekeeping, assistance with older children, making meals, laundry, and baby-care basics, including teaching you how to care for your new baby and help with breastfeeding. Each postpartum doula can help you decide what your greatest needs are and figure out how to get you these services quickly and efficiently. Most families use a postpartum doula from when the new baby comes home until around three months of age. Some doulas work several hours a day for several days a week, while others come just one day a week. It really is tailored to your needs.

I would encourage you to interview the postpartum doulas in your area. See what services they provide and how they might help your family. Ask other families with new babies if they can recommend someone.

Getting help in the postpartum period is a must. Whether you have personal or professional help, begin your planning early. This will help ensure the smoothest transition possible.

ELSEWHERE ON THE WEB

▸ Finding a professional postpartum doula isn't hard. I'd recommend you look at DONA International's Web site (www.dona.org) for their doula finder. This organization actually trains and certifies people to be able to help in the postpartum period. A postpartum doula can help you make sure that the first weeks and months of your baby's life aren't as stressful as they would be if you tried to do everything alone. Sometimes it's just nice to have an experienced pair of hands around to help out.

Get Linked

From prenatal bonding to holding your baby for the first time, there is a lot to learn for both parents. Trying to keep your family on an even keel after a birth doesn't have to be a horrible thing. Planning ahead by learning is always best, so here are some links to help you and dad-to-be.

FOR FATHERS ONLY

Here's a source of basic pregnancy information for dads, including birth stories by dads and information on making the most of your pregnancy and postpartum.

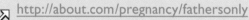 http://about.com/pregnancy/fathersonly

GETTING DAD INVOLVED IN PREGNANCY

Is he looking for great ways to show he cares? Here are some quick and easy ways to be an involved dad when it comes to pregnancy.

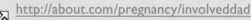 http://about.com/pregnancy/involveddad

BABY CARE COURSE

Dad-to-be can ease his fears of caring for a new baby by learning the basics. This e-mail course covers basics like baths for baby, diapering, swaddling, and burping.

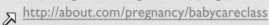 http://about.com/pregnancy/babycareclass

Chapter 15

Multiple Blessings

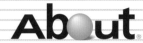

The Discovery: More Than One!

Congratulations! You're in for a wild ride. The shock of finding out that there is more than one baby on the way can be immense. Whether you find out early in your pregnancy or later, the moment is one you will never forget.

Most people will find out they are expecting multiples via an ultrasound. Sometimes you get this news very early on, as in around six or seven weeks into your pregnancy. Perhaps you were seen for bleeding or had high hCG levels that your practitioner wanted to check out. If you had fertility treatments, you will usually have an early ultrasound done as a check before sending you out for pregnancy care.

The benefits of finding out early are numerous. It means that you have more time to learn and plan for your babies. It also gives you a head start on taking extra care with your nutrition, health, and prenatal care.

Surprise! The other time you're likely find out you're having multiples is during an ultrasound later in pregnancy. Maybe you're having some signs that there is more than one baby in there, like any of these:

- Your uterine measurements are large for your pregnancy.
- You feel a lot of movement, more than one baby could make.
- You have very severe morning sickness.
- Your lab work numbers don't make sense, such as AFP testing or others.

While many people would expect you to be overjoyed to find out that multiples are on the way, that is not always the case. Remember this is very unusual news for most families. Normal reactions to finding out you're having multiples vary from feelings of excitement to being overwhelmed, to tears and even fear.

Don't be concerned if your first thought isn't a positive one. Once the initial haze wears off, you'll have plenty of time for the reality to sink in. This is when the hard work of preparing for multiples begins.

You may want to know how this happened. How did you get so lucky as to have twins? Generally speaking, the natural rate of twins is about one in ninety births. Since the 1980s, that number has gone up for a variety of reasons, including fertility treatments and the number of women over thirty-five who are giving birth. You are also more likely to conceive twins if you have a maternal family history of twins, got pregnant while breastfeeding, or were overweight when you got pregnant.

Identical or fraternal? This question will start early on, in fact, usually as soon as you announce your pregnancy. During early

ELSEWHERE ON THE WEB

▶ When I found out that twins were on the way, I needed information and support. One of the best things I did was to contact my local Mothers of Twins club. They had a great program set up to help educate me, support me, and provide me with the tools I needed to get through my twin pregnancy. Find your local club on the Web through the National Organization of Mothers of Twins Clubs, at www.nomotc.org.

pregnancy there are not always good ways to tell if your babies are monozygotic (identical) or dizygotic (fraternal).

Sometimes early ultrasounds can say that your babies share an amnion or that there are two separate placentas, but ultrasound is not always done early on to make this apparent. Later in pregnancy, if you can determine that you are carrying a boy and a girl, then you will know your babies are dizygotic.

Sometimes genetic testing is the only way to know for sure if your babies are monozygotic or dizygotic. There might be guesses based on placentas or looks, but remember these are not always accurate. Some twins who look identical are really just similar-looking siblings. Even if you did in vitro fertilization and returned only two embryos, you could still have monozygotic twins (or triplets). Be sure to ask your doctor or midwife what testing can be done to help you if you desire this knowledge.

Wanting to know this information is perfectly normal. While some parents may want to know for curiosity reasons, there may be times later in life when knowing is important, as in some medical situations. Not knowing is not harmful, and the information can be determined at any point down the road, not just at birth.

Multiply the Pregnancy Changes

During the first trimester, the rate of growth of your multiples is just like that of other singleton babies. At about thirty weeks of gestation, the rate of growth for multiples tends to slow. This is because their bodies put more energy into lung development. Since 60 percent of twins are born before 36 weeks, earlier lung development is a good thing for your babies.

Normal pregnancy symptoms may be exacerbated because of more babies. This means that morning sickness may be more frequent or last longer. You may start to feel aches

ELSEWHERE ON THE WEB

▶ There are DNA testing kits that you can order to test your multiples after they are born to see whether they are identical or fraternal. My husband and I suffered from a case of curiosity, so we did it when our twins were three weeks old. These are simple kits done by swabbing your baby's cheek. To learn more about the process, see www .proactivegenetics.com and www.affiliatedgenetics.com.

and pains of pregnancy earlier in your pregnancy as well. There is no reason that you can't deal with these symptoms the same way a singleton mom would.

Did you know that the size of your uterus with twins at twenty-eight weeks is the same size as someone else's 40-week size uterus? That is probably one of the most staggering facts I read when expecting my twins. For fun be sure to take waist measurements and to keep a record of how big your uterus gets. Pictures, no matter how tired you are, are also recommended for good fun!

One of the best pieces of advice I have for a mother of multiples is to rest. Instituting a rest period in every day, early on, even before I really needed it, helped me tremendously. Several women have said that their practitioners also recommended this as the best way to avoid bed rest in a multiple pregnancy.

I came home every day after work and grabbed a snack on my way to lie down in bed. Sometimes I would use the time to nap or read. The older kids liked to join me, but they quickly learned it was quiet time. Sometimes we'd read together or play baby kicking games with the babies. One of our daughters loved to play guessing games about baby names. This quickly became a sweet and wonderful time I looked forward to every day. As my pregnancy got further along, I rested for longer times. I tried to lie down for at least twenty or thirty minutes each day.

With a multiple pregnancy, you are also at greater risk for certain pregnancy complications. Some of these could occur in any pregnancy, and some are specific to multiples only. These may include the following:

- Preterm labor
- High blood pressure
- Twin-to-twin transfusion syndrome (TTTS)
- Monoamniotic-monochorinoic twins

▶ Your regular pregnancy books will only cover part of what you need now! *When You're Expecting Twins, Triplets or Quads,* by Barbara Luke, is a great source of comfort. I liked reading what other moms had to say about being pregnant with multiples, as well as the normally sane advice from a scientist. This book was always open on my nightstand.

- Diabetes
- Placental issues
- Heart problems
- Postpartum bleeding

Twin-to-twin transfusion syndrome (TTTS) involves communication between the placentas that causes one twin to receive too much blood (possibly leading to heart failure), while the other twin suffers from anemia.

Monoamniotic-monochorinoic twins share a single amnion and a single chorion, leading to the drastic problem of potential cord entanglement.

Nutrition is even more important for multiples. A link has been found between your nutritional status and how long your gestation is likely to be. Try thinking of every meal and snack as time you're not spending in the neonatal intensive care unit (NICU). In fact, the sooner you gain weight, the better off you are, even if you do have the babies early.

This is because the baby has gained more weight prior to that point based on your nutritional status. Try to gain twenty-five pounds by week 20 gestation for twins, thirty-five pounds for triplets, and forty-five pounds for quadruplets. By week 38, you should have gained between forty and fifty-six pounds for twins, fifty-eight and seventy-five pounds for triplets, and seventy to eighty pounds for quadruplets, This is according to Dr. Barbara Luke, a professor of obstetrics and gynecology and a nutritionist from The University of Michigan's Multiples Clinic.

Obviously the more babies you have in your uterus, the more calories you will need. Dr. Luke's recommendation is that you eat 176 grams of protein for twins, 200 for triplets, and 225 for

ASK YOUR GUIDE

Will I have restrictions on everything?

▶ Generally speaking, you are likely to have restrictions on nearly everything in your life with a multiple pregnancy. Things like your sex life or travel will be restricted depending on your health, the health of the babies, and where you are in your pregnancy. Taking a rest period every day early on can help you avoid or delay severe restrictions later.

quadruplets. This can be very hard to do, especially when you may not feel like eating.

I found switching to whole milk products helped add protein, as did snacking on hard-boiled eggs. There were days my husband would make me breakfast of a fruit smoothie with protein powder. Other mothers suggest adding cheese to things like spaghetti, sandwiches, and scrambled eggs. Nuts are easy to carry and high in protein for quick and easy snacks.

Preterm labor is more likely in multiple pregnancy. Remember that 60 percent of twins are born before week 36 of pregnancy. That percentage rate goes up for every additional baby in your uterus.

During your pregnancy you will be monitored for signs of preterm labor. (For a refresher course on possible complications in pregnancy, including preterm labor, see Chapter 8.) One of the additional ways that a multiple pregnancy is monitored is via ultrasound. You will have additional ultrasounds to screen for appropriate growth in your babies, placental development, position of the babies, and the length of your cervix.

The length of your cervix will be measured at every ultrasound. Typically you will have monthly ultrasounds beginning between eighteen and twenty weeks and bi-weekly or weekly ultrasounds after twenty-eight weeks, depending on your practitioner and your pregnancy. If your practitioner sees signs of your cervix opening prematurely (with or without contractions) or signs that one or more of your babies isn't growing well, you may be asked to go on bed rest.

While bed rest as a matter of routine is not beneficial, if you are having contractions or your cervix is dilating, bed rest can help reduce the strain on your cervix. It can also wind up being a break to stop and catch your breath and get your life in order. The power

TOOLS YOU NEED

▶ With the weight of more than one baby and the additional strains on your back, belly, and cervix, you need a lift. The use of a support device, like a Prenatal Cradle, can really help you feel more comfortable during your pregnancy. Using a full-body device seems to work best for most mothers; the belly-only support is just too light for multiple babies.

of positive thinking can help you survive bed rest as well as help you maintain a sense of calm.

How Labor Works with More Than One Baby

Most women are concerned about labor. That concern grows when there is more than one baby—and rightfully so. Having a normal birth with twins is usually more difficult, and more of the factors are out of your control.

You should begin planning for your labor and birth as soon as possible; the first trimester is not too early. You will want to interview your chosen practitioner again to ask him your many twin or higher-order multiple-related questions, including these:

- Do you do multiples in your practice?
- What experience do you have with multiples?
- Do you have a high-risk practice to refer me to if I should need it?
- Do you deliver the second baby breech or try to convert the baby to vertex?
- Can I have my twins in the regular labor room?
- If I have a vaginal birth in the operating room, can I still use the labor bed?
- Do you impose regular time limits between babies?
- What is your policy on the length of gestation for twins? Triplets? More?
- Do you routinely use forceps or vacuum extraction for a second twin?
- What is your belief about pain medication for a vaginal twin birth?
- If the babies are born healthy, can they stay in the room after birth?

ELSEWHERE ON THE WEB

▶ If you're looking for support from others who have been there, the Internet is a great resource. There are many sites where parents of multiples gather to have discussions about any topic related to multiples. One such site I frequented was the AP Multiples Yahoo Group (http://groups.yahoo.com/group/apmultiples). Here I could ask questions, talk to other parents, read birth stories, and get parenting advice from others who had been there.

You should really consider taking a special class designed just for parents of multiples. This is usually a one-time class that is a nice addition to a regular childbirth class. You should also try to arrange a tour of the NICU along with the hospital during a class or at an appointment with your practitioner.

This childbirth class will help you think of questions to ask your birth team. It will also go over all the possibilities for giving birth to multiples. It should cover vaginal birth, cesarean birth, breastfeeding, and caring for a baby in the NICU. There may be classes like this offered by private instructors, your local Mothers of Twins Club, or at the hospital near you.

Vaginal birth is possible with multiples. The American College of Obstetricians and Gynecologists (ACOG) recommends a vaginal birth as long as the baby closest to your cervix is vertex. The first baby is in this head-down position in more than 80 percent of pregnancies when labor starts.

During labor you may be monitored more closely, though unless you are being induced, are on certain medications, or have something questionable going on, you can still use intermittent monitoring for your babies. (See Chapter 10 for information on labor interventions.) You will have a belt for a contractions monitor, as well as a belt for each baby. That makes three belts for twins, four belts for triplets, and so on.

Labor with multiples is usually very much like laboring with a single baby. Sometimes, because of the larger size of the uterus, the contractions are not as effective. This may or may not matter depending on the length of your cervix. You should be allowed to move around and assume positions for labor as with any other labor.

Once your cervix is fully dilated, you will be allowed to push or instructed to push. Recent studies have shown that pushing

▶ Think about how you feel about an unmedicated birth. If you had previously been planning to not have medications, how does having multiples affect this decision? Sometimes as a compromise, a practitioner might suggest that you have an epidural catheter placed, but not used. That way you can labor without medication and use the epidural only if it is needed for an emergency situation. If you want an unmedicated birth, you can have that experience with a backup plan.

when you feel like it is best, but if you have an epidural, you may need some guidance for the first baby. You may assume positions that are comfortable during pushing. You are still likely to push for awhile with most first pregnancies and less with subsequent pregnancies. I personally wound up pushing for a bit longer than with my previous pregnancies.

The birth of the first baby goes just like any other singleton. Once the baby is born, she will be placed on your abdomen or in your arms, unless she needs special help. This is where vaginal birth really gets different for moms of multiples.

Your mind is split between the baby just born and the one about to be born, and so is your husband's. Your practitioner and assistants are watching your first baby and monitoring what is going on with your second baby. There can be anywhere from minutes to hours between babies. As long as the second baby is doing well, there is no reason to hurry things along.

During your wait, you may have some time to get to know your first baby. You can hold your baby and love her. Do everything you imagined in holding your new baby. After our first daughter was born, I cried and held her. I told her to enjoy being the youngest child because it wasn't going to last long. And twenty-three minutes later, there came her sister.

If you find that holding your firstborn baby is hard because you are anxious for the next baby or the pushing yet to come, consider letting Dad hold the baby and get support from your doula for a while.

You will also likely be monitored with an ultrasound to see the position of the next baby. Sometimes the breech or transverse baby, suddenly given a ton of space, will spontaneously turn head down before being born. Some practitioners choose to help the baby turn, while others prefer to have her born breech.

The birth of the second baby is usually a bit more worrisome for your practitioners. They will be monitoring position and health while waiting for your cervix to dilate again, if your cervix went down in dilation, or for contractions to resume. Sometimes you can nurse your first baby to get contractions going again and not need Pitocin.

During the second birth, your doctor or midwife may decide that additional help is needed. This may mean an episiotomy, a manual version (turning baby into a more favorable position), breech extraction (pulling the baby out by his feet) or other methods to help encourage baby to come down and out.

Once both babies are born, you will nearly be finished with labor. All that is left now is to push out the placentas. These usually come within thirty minutes after the babies are born. They may come together, having grown together in the uterus; there may be only one; or they may come separately. The birth of the placentas is usually not painful for you. I always tell moms that there are no bones in these, which make them much easier to birth!

Cesarean section is done for 50 percent of twin births.

Some of these may be for valid medical reasons, but other times it is purely the practitioner's preference to deliver all twins or multiples in this manner. This is where a good relationship and knowledge of your practitioner come in very handy.

The most common reason to have a scheduled cesarean for multiples is that the baby closest to the cervix is not in a head-down position. This happens in about 20 percent of all multiples. The other reasons for cesarean section are the same as in singleton births:

- Placenta previa
- Placental abruption
- Pregnancy-induced hypertension

BEFORE YOUR APPOINTMENT

▶ Pack your labor bags early in pregnancy with multiples, around twenty-eight weeks to be exact. Since you never know when your babies may be born, be prepared! One mom kept the basics by the door, so that all she had to do was add her toothbrush should she need it. She said she felt like it warded off the demon of preterm labor, and gratefully, she didn't have to touch the bag until she was thirty-eight weeks pregnant.

- Active herpes
- Fetal distress
- Other labor complications

If you have a scheduled cesarean birth, it will usually be planned for week 37 or 38 of pregnancy. Sometimes you go into labor prior to your scheduled surgery, or your water breaks. If that happens to you, you will be admitted for the surgery immediately at that point.

The surgery itself is very similar to the cesarean surgery for a singleton. (See Chapter 11.) Usually your babies will be born within a minute or two of each other. Then the placentas are delivered. If the babies are doing well, they should be allowed to stay with you in the operating room.

Here's an interesting note about birth order. In pregnancy Baby A is the name for the baby closest to your cervix. In a cesarean birth, the first baby out is called Baby A. This is not always the baby closest to your cervix. If you had a baby name picked out for the lowest-in-the-pelvis baby, make sure you ask your surgeon who is really whom at birth.

Occasionally you have a vaginal birth and a cesarean. This happens about 4 percent of the time with twins. The first baby is born vaginally, and the second twin is not able to be born that way. This reason is usually something more of an emergency, like a cord prolapse or a placental abruption or fetal distress, rather than positioning. A cesarean is then done to birth that twin or other multiple.

The good news about this is that because of the labor, your baby is better prepared for life outside the uterus. He will usually have a smoother recovery than if you had chosen a scheduled cesarean for your birth.

ASK YOUR GUIDE

If I had a previous cesarean, can I now have a vaginal birth?

▶ This is more a question that is determined by your practitioner's preference, as there is no reason not to have a trial of labor or vaginal birth with twins if all other factors are normal. Be sure to ask your doctor to look at the medical literature with you if you have questions.

The immediate postpartum will be watchful. You and your babies will be monitored carefully for any signs of problems or distress. If your babies are term or near term and are doing well, they will most likely be with you in the recovery and postpartum period. You can decide if you wish them to go to the well newborn nursery for baths or choose to hold them yourselves.

Since you are at a greater risk of some postpartum complications, including postpartum hemorrhage, you will be monitored very carefully in recovery. This is true whether you had a vaginal birth or a cesarean. This is because the extra stretching in the uterus may make it more difficult for your uterus to control its own bleeding. Nursing your babies can help stave off any bleeding problems by releasing your body's own hormonal defense—oxytocin.

Spend these first few hours holding your babies. Look at their bodies, snuggle with them, and simply enjoy them. You have worked very hard to get to this point.

If your babies are ill, ask to be taken to them. You may be asked to wait until you are out of your immediate postpartum period or until they have been stabilized in the NICU or other nursery. Most hospitals can provide you with instant photographs of the babies even if you and the babies cannot be together. Consider sending your husband or doula to stay with the babies or to relay news about them to you.

Coping with Multiples at Home and on the Go

The day when your babies come home can be a time of great excitement. Sometimes you may have one baby come home before the other, or you may be lucky enough to have them come home together. No matter when your babies come home, there is a time of learning and preparation. Being easy on yourself and getting a few of the basics down will help ease this transition.

Get to know your babies. This might seem like a huge task with double the baby, but it is doable. The first part of this is learning how to tell your babies apart. This terrified me at first. You can paint a toenail, use special clothing, or even have bracelets made for your babies. This not only helps you, but it helps others as well.

I remember when Owen and Clara were just tiny and I was crying because everyone could tell them apart except for me. What kind of mother did that make me? It turns out I was a fine mother, but bracelets helped keep me sane.

Learn to see the babies both as individuals and as a set. Obviously learning them as a set can come more easily and naturally. Try to have some one-on-one time with each baby every day. This is done easily during feeding, bathing, or even diapering times. This also encourages others to spend alone time with your babies.

Get help at home. Probably one of the easiest things to do wrong with multiples is to not accept help. There are many people who would be more than willing to help you and your family if you would let them.

Do not try to be supermom and do everything yourself. Having one baby is hard, and I'd venture to guess most mothers of multiples would tell you that for every baby you add, there is more than a 100-percent increase in the workload, simply because of the extra time and effort involved in caring for the babies. Your help can be as simple as utilizing grandparents or friends.

When people call to say they are coming to visit, they usually ask if they can bring something. Tell them what they can bring. Ask for a meal, even if you freeze it. Tell them you're running low on laundry detergent or toilet paper. They can't read your mind when it comes to what you need. So be specific and allow them to help. One of the things we often forget about when getting help is how good it feels

TOOLS YOU NEED

▶ *Mothering Multiples,* by Karen Kerkoff Gromada, a mother of twins and a lactation consultant, is the answer to your postbirth needs. Reading it prior to the birth of your babies is very helpful, and the parenting and breastfeeding advice is very down to earth and practical. In addition to the everyday help, there is also a great section on babies who need special care and hospitalization.

to be able to help others. By accepting help, you are allowing your friends and family to feel really good about helping you.

Perhaps you don't have a lot of family or friends around to help you. Don't sweat it. Here are some other places to look for help:

- Your place of worship
- Your neighbors
- Local multiples club
- Babysitters
- Postpartum doulas

A postpartum doula is an especially great idea for mothers of multiples. Since they are trained to help keep the house running and give you any needed baby advice, you get twice your money's worth in these gems. Need breastfeeding advice? No problem. Need dinner for the family? She's got that covered, too.

Getting out of the house will help you keep your sanity. It is not so easy to do with more than one baby. But even a short time out of the house will help you maintain your sanity.

We spent a lot of time walking around our neighborhood after the girls were born. At first we used one stroller that laid all the way back to take the girls on walks. They snuggled next to one another and I got to stretch and exercise a bit. It was also nice to have adult conversations with the neighbors, no matter how brief.

Taking babies out with two cars seats can be a bit more daunting. I highly recommend keeping the diaper bag packed and a stash of emergency clothes and diapers in the vehicle. This allows you to walk out the door quickly with your normal diaper bag, but not flip out if you go through all the supplies that you had with you.

I had a great double stroller that allowed my car seats to snap right into the stroller. This was quick and easy and I didn't have to

WHAT'S HOT

▶ As soon as you find out you're expecting multiples, call your insurance company. Tell them that you need a case manager with experience with multiples, if possible, assigned to your case. This person will be your go-to person for insurance-related questions about your care and the care of your babies. Even if you don't require extensive hospitalization of either of the twins, there can be glitches. One pharmacy constantly gets denials for one of our twin's medicine if we try to fill identical prescriptions on the same day. The reason? They share a birthday.

take each baby out of the car seat. This worked well for over a year.

For trips out when they weren't to be in car seats, I truly enjoyed the sling. My husband also loved to carry the babies around this way. Unlike front carriers, a sling can hold two tiny babies together. You can also wear two slings, like the Maya Wrap, for older babies. My girls loved this closeness, and I loved having my hands free to shop, hold older kids' hands, or do whatever I needed to do.

Don't hesitate to ask for help when you go out. Consider a quick lunch out every week or so if you can swing it. Bring a friend to help, and enjoy going out with the babies. The worst part of taking out multiples is the questions you get asked. So be prepared to deal with any number of these questions or comments:

- Are they twins?
- Are they identical or fraternal?
- How do you tell them apart?
- Did you take fertility drugs?
- I wish I had twins.
- I'm glad they're yours and not mine.

Well meaning or not, these questions and comments can get a bit old. There are some T-shirts with answers to these questions available. One mom I know actually made a sign for her stroller with the answers obvious to everyone.

Having multiples or babies in general is a learning experience but a delightful one for most. The joy of raising your child and learning to care for him is a satisfying, but difficult job. Looking back at the end of a pregnancy or at a first birthday at how far you have come with your little one will really amaze you. Enjoy your babies!

BEFORE YOUR APPOINTMENT

▶ Keeping a daily log for each of the babies can help you keep the details straight in your now very hectic life. You might believe you'll remember whose diaper you changed or who nursed when, but chances are you will either forget. A daily record of who nursed which side, how long, dirty and wet diapers, and maybe even a space for medication can be very helpful. Take this with you to the pediatrician so she can see how the days go for you and offer any help.

Get Linked

Having multiples can be frightening and wonderful all in the same breath. Learning all you can and planning ahead will help you keep your cool and enjoy as much of the journey as you can. The following links are gathered to help you accomplish that goal.

MULTIPLE PREGNANCY

So, you're expecting multiples? These links will help you figure out what to do from the positive pregnancy test, the regular physical exams, ultrasounds, testing, bringing your babies home, and much more!

 http://about.com/pregnancy/multiples

**TWINS AND MULTIPLES
ULTRASOUND
AND BELLY GALLERY**

In this gallery guide, you'll find areas for multiple ultrasound photos as well as the bellies of mothers carrying multiples from different stages in pregnancy. You can compare them to photos of singleton moms just to see how very different being pregnant with more than one can be.

 http://about.com/pregnancy/pregnancygallery

MULTIPLE BIRTH STORIES

Interested in reading about how others families gave birth to their multiples? Here you can read about vaginal births, cesareans, and all the details of the labor and birth. Some even talk a bit about the postpartum life with two or more babies. If you're interested, you can submit your stories, too.

 http://about.com/pregnancy/multiplestories

Appendix A

Glossary

amnioinfusion

A way to put fluids into the uterus via a catheter, used in labor to decrease meconium staining and rehydrate the uterus.

amnion

The inner layer of the amniotic sac that encloses the baby in the uterus.

amniotic fluid

The fluid that surrounds the baby in the uterus, made up mostly of fetal urine.

amniotomy

Artificial breaking of the bag of waters (amniotic sac) surrounding the baby.

anemia

Iron deficiency treated with diet and supplements.

areola

The darker portion of the breast.

artificial baby milk

Commercially produced cow milk or soy-based product (also known as formula) designed to imitate human breast milk. Though science has not been able to do this with any real success, it is consumable by infants.

auscultation

Listening to the baby using a stethoscope or fetoscope—no machines.

basal thermometer

A device to measure body temperature in tenths of degrees to detect small changes in a woman's temperature to help pinpoint ovulation.

bilirubin

Byproduct of the breakdown of red blood cells.

blastocyst

Early stage of development in a baby.

blighted ovum

An ovum that fails to fully develop, ending in pregnancy loss.

bloody show

Slight bloody discharge from the vagina that usually precedes labor by a few days to weeks as the cervix begins to open.

breech

When the part nearest the cervix is the buttocks of the baby, he is said to be breech.

breech extraction

In a twin birth, this refers to the pulling of the baby out by his feet to assist in the birth.

cerclage

Sutures placed in the cervix to prevent its premature opening.

certified nurse midwife (CNM)

A nurse who has taken additional training in normal pregnancy, birth, and postpartum and well-woman care.

cervical mucous

Mucous that helps at conception, leaving the body from the cervix.

cervix
The mouth of the uterus, which opens into the vagina.

cesarean section
Birth by which the baby is removed via a surgical opening in the abdomen.

cholasma
Dark pigmentation, usually found on the face, due to hormones in pregnancy.

chorion
The outer layer of the amniotic sac, which lines the uterus during pregnancy.

colostrum
Golden-colored premilk substance that is nutrient-dense and packed with antibodies for the baby.

congenital anomaly
A malformation of the baby that developed prior to birth.

cord prolapse
Where the umbilical cord comes down into the opening of the cervix before the baby. This is an emergency situation, usually requiring a cesarean delivery.

counterpressure
Direct pressure to the lower back, usually during labor, to aid in pain relief.

dilate
The act of the opening of the cervix.

dilation and curettage (D&C)
A surgical procedure where the cervix is dilated and the contents of the uterus are removed.

directed bearing down
Being told when to push during the second stage of labor.

dizygotic
Twins that come from separate eggs, also called fraternal twins.

Doppler
Hand-held device used to listen to the baby's heartbeat in pregnancy.

doula
A trained professional in labor who helps families in the pregnancy, birth, and postpartum period.

dystocia
Abnormal pattern to labor.

ectopic pregnancy (tubal pregnancy)
A pregnancy that implants someplace other than the uterus, like the cervix, fallopian tube, abdomen, etc.

efface
The thinning of the cervix.

embryo
Stage of fetal development between blastocyst and fetus.

emergency cesarean
Surgical, abdominal birth done usually within minutes of the decision for surgery to save the life of mother or baby. Not planned in advance.

engorgement
An overabundant breast milk supply that can cause discomfort in the mother, usually in the first week of baby's life.

endometrial lining
The lining of the uterus where the fertilized egg implants.

epidural anesthesia
A regional form of numbing that takes away painful sensation from your nipples to your knees.

episiotomy

A surgical cut made in the perineum to facilitate the birth.

external fetal monitoring

A device used to monitor baby's heart rate during labor, using ultrasound and external belts.

fallopian tubes

The parts of the uterine anatomy that attach the uterus to the ovaries.

female factor infertility

Infertility that is traced back to problems with the female.

fertile mucous

Discharge from the cervix that is conducive to conception.

fetal alcohol syndrome (FAS)

Severe problems in the baby caused by maternal drinking both in mental and physical development and abilities.

fetal alcohol effects (FAE)

Lower-level problems in the way of physical and/or deformities/disabilities caused by maternal drinking in pregnancy.

fetal distress

Nonreassuring fetal heart tones, usually in labor.

fetal fibronectin

A protein found in the placenta, used to predict preterm delivery.

fetal growth restriction

When the baby does not grow as expected due to some other problem with the pregnancy, baby, or mother.

fetal heart tones

Your baby's heart rate during pregnancy as heard by Doppler, fetoscope, etc.

fetal kick counts

A way to monitor the baby's health by keeping count of perceptible movements.

fetoscope

A special stethoscope designed specifically for pregnant women.

fetus

Period of baby's development after 12 weeks, after the embryonic stage.

fundal height

Measurement from the top of your uterus to your pubic bone, taken at your prenatal appointments.

general anesthesia

A type of anesthesia used for surgery, in which a sleeplike state is induced.

gestational diabetes

A diabetic condition of pregnancy.

glucose tolerance testing

A test given during pregnancy to test for the presence of gestational diabetes.

group B strep

A type of infection that is the leading cause of blood infection and meningitis in newborns.

hemorrhoids

Varicose veins in the rectum.

heartburn

When stomach acid backs up into the esophagus, causing pain.

hCG

Human chorionic gonadotropin, the hormone produced in pregnancy and measured in pregnancy tests.

hyperemesis gravidarum

Severe version of morning sickness usually leading to dehydration and potential hospitalization.

incompetent cervix

A weak cervix that can dilate too early, causing preterm labor or even stillbirth due to early birth.

induction of labor

Artificial means are used to create contractions and hopefully labor to end in the birth of your baby.

infertility

The inability to have a baby after a year of trying to conceive with timed intercourse and no birth control use.

internal uterine pressure catheter (IUPC)

A device used to measure exact amounts of pressure inside the uterus during labor.

intracytoplasmic sperm injection (ICSI)

A single sperm is placed inside a single egg with a special needle, during the IVF procedure.

intrauterine growth restriction

See fetal growth restriction.

intrauterine insemination (IUI)

A fertility treatment in which sperm is placed inside a small catheter and then delivered directly to the uterus.

intravenous (IV)

A needle is used to insert a small plastic catheter to allow the administration of medications or fluids into a vein in your body.

in vitro fertilization (IVF)

Fertility treatment in which the sperm and egg are joined in a Petri dish and the resulting embryos are placed back inside the uterus.

lanugo

Downy hair that covers the baby during most of the pregnancy.

laparoscopy

Form of surgery involving several small incisions.

laparotomy

Abdominal surgery using a small incision on the lower abdomen.

linea negra

A dark line that can extend down the center of your abdomen in pregnancy due to hormones.

lochia

Normal postpartum bleeding as the uterus heals.

maternal fetal medicine specialist (MFM/perinatologist)

Physician who specializes in high-risk pregnancy and birth.

male factor infertility

Fertility problem directly related to the male in the partnership.

manual extraction

Where a baby is removed from the uterus using the hands, usually in a twin birth. See breech extraction.

menstrual cycle

The cycle of hormonal events that lead to ovulation and menstruation.

methotrexate

Medication used to treat ectopic pregnancy without surgery.

miscarriage

The end of a pregnancy prior to 20 weeks of gestation due to problems with the baby or the pregnancy.

monozygotic

Twins formed from the splitting of a single egg, also known as identical twins.

Montgomery tubercles

Small glands that are raised on the areola during pregnancy.

morning sickness

Feelings of nausea and vomiting that accompany pregnancy, more often in the early weeks, probably due to hormonal changes.

neonatal intensive care unit (NICU)

The highest level of nursery care available for the sickest infants, particularly babies who are born prematurely.

neural tube defects

Congenital anomalies that are of the neural tube, such as spina bifida or anencephaly.

nursing pad

Small pad of cotton, washable or disposable, used to catch extra breast milk that may leak.

obstetrician (OB)

Physician specializing in pregnancy.

oligohydramnios

A syndrome of low amniotic fluid levels.

ovaries

Gonads of the females that produce the eggs for fertilization in ovulation.

ovulation

Process of releasing an egg during the menstrual cycle.

ovulation induction

The use of medication to induce or supplement ovulation.

ovulation prediction kit (OPK)

At home medical kit used to detect hormones indicating ovulation is about to occur. Used for trying to get pregnant.

ovum

An egg prior to fertilization.

oxytocin

Hormone that helps the process of labor start and continue, as well as aid breast milk production and letdown.

period

The menstrual flow of the menstrual cycle.

Pitocin

Artificial or synthetic form of the hormone oxytocin used to induce or augment contractions in labor.

placenta abruption

Where the placenta tears off the wall of the uterus prior to birth, creating a life-threatening situation.

placenta previa

Condition in which the placenta grows near or covers the cervix.

polyhydramnios

Condition of overproduction of amniotic fluid.

pregnancy-induced hypertension (PIH)

Condition of high blood pressure in pregnancy.

premature birth

When birth occurs before 37 weeks in a singleton pregnancy.

preterm labor

Where labor ensues prior to 37 weeks of pregnancy; can be treated to prevent preterm birth.

primary cesarean rate

Rate of first-time surgical births, this does not include women having repeat cesareans.

quickening

When you first feel your baby move.

recovery room

A special room near the operating room, for the immediate time period after surgery when you will need closer observation.

reproductive endocrinologist

Physician who specializes in the diagnosis and treatment of infertility.

Rh factor

Antigen present or not present in your blood.

rice sock

A sock filled with plain white rice, used for heat therapy in pregnancy and labor.

saline lock

An IV port is placed in case it is needed for emergency, but not connected to any tubing or wires.

scheduled cesarean

A surgical, abdominal birth planned before labor and begins at a specified time and place.

spontaneous bearing down

Listening to one's body to push.

station

 The relationship of the baby to the mother's pelvis, measures from –5 to +5.

stillbirth

The death of a baby after 20 weeks of pregnancy but prior to birth.

stress tests

A fetal test where a small amount of medication is given to cause contractions to see if the baby can tolerate the stress of labor.

stretch marks

Areas where the skin breaks down, usually on the abdomen.

Trendelenberg position

Lying with the feet above the head to prevent preterm birth.

twin-to-twin transfusion syndrome (TTTS)

In monozygotic twins, where there is connection between the placentas so that one twin gives more blood to the other baby causing one baby to suffer from heart failure and the other from severe anemia.

ultrasound

Sound waves used to produce images of the baby while you are still pregnant.

unexplained infertility

A situation in which a couple cannot get pregnant, but no reason is found.

unscheduled cesarean

A surgical, abdominal birth done during labor, that was not planned in advance, nor is it an emergency.

uterus

Also known as the womb, this organ expands to accommodate the growing pregnancy and shrinks back down after the birth.

vertex

When the baby is in a head-down position.

Appendix B

Pregnancy Month by Month

Prepregnancy

Things for Dad to do before getting pregnant:
- ○ Have a complete physical exam.
- ○ Quit smoking.
- ○ Check your insurance for maternity coverage.
- ○ Attend prepregnancy visits with your partner.
- ○ Find out about paternity leave at your work.

Things for Mom to do before getting pregnant:
- ○ Get a prepregnancy physical.
- ○ Interview potential practitioners.
- ○ Get to know your cycle to help you get pregnant faster.
- ○ Get healthy (quit smoking, etc.).
- ○ Take a prepregnancy class if available.

FIRST TRIMESTER

First Month
Mother
- You are not pregnant as this month begins.
- You will have your last period.
- After ovulation, the egg and sperm meet and begin the journey to the uterus.
- Toward the end of the month, you may start to suspect you are pregnant.

Baby
- Your baby is conceived.
- The blastocyst implants in the uterus.
- The yolk sac will sustain your pregnancy until the placenta takes over.
- Your baby will measure between 1 and 2 mm by the end of this month.

Things to do this month:
- ○ Take prenatal or multivitamins as you plan for pregnancy.
- ○ Track your cycle to predict ovulation to time when you are most likely to conceive.
- ○ Act pregnant when it comes to alcohol and other medications/drugs.
- ○ Be sure to take care of your body with healthy food and exercise.

Second Month
Mother
- You should have a positive pregnancy test by blood or urine.
- You may begin to have nausea and vomiting.
- Fatigue is likely to set in.
- Your lower abdomen may feel heavy, but you are unlikely to show.

Baby

- Your baby's heart begins to beat this month.
- The beginnings of the liver, pancreas, lungs, and stomach are evident.
- Finger and toe rays are present.
- Your baby is now measuring between 8 and 11 mm from head to bottom, known as crown-to-rump length (CRL).

Things to do this month:

- ○ Interview and select a midwife or doctor.
- ○ Double-check your maternity benefits and your patient rights and responsibilities.
- ○ Take an early pregnancy class.
- ○ Start a journal or a scrapbook.
- ○ Start to take pictures and measurements of your belly monthly.

Third Month

Mother

- May feel better toward the end of this month.
- May feel bloated as uterus rises out of pelvis at the end of the month.
- Pregnancy symptoms continue, like morning sickness, fatigue, and heartburn.
- Breathing rate increases.
- Breast changes may include fuller breasts, bigger and darker areolas.

Baby

- Baby moves spontaneously.
- Bones begin to harden.
- Eyes are large and open, with no eyelids.
- Baby weighs about 14 grams and is approximately 3.54 inches in total length.

Things to do this month:

- ○ Have you had your first prenatal visit? Try scheduling a couple ahead to get the best times and dates for your schedule.
- ○ Consider early prenatal tests like nuchal fold scan, amniocentesis, or CVS.
- ○ Visit birth centers and hospitals for tours and interviews.
- ○ If you haven't shared your good news, you may consider doing so now.

SECOND TRIMESTER

Fourth Month

Mother

- Placenta has taken over production of pregnancy hormones.
- Your belly may begin to show.
- You probably feel a lot better than last month.
- Heart is working harder than usual because of extra blood volume.

Baby

- Makes some of its own insulin and bile.
- Urinates into amniotic fluid every forty-five minutes or so.
- Heart pumps about twenty-five quarts of blood a day.
- Your baby is about 3 ounces (85 grams) and 6.3 inches (16 cm).

Things to do this month:

- ○ Make decisions about prenatal testing like AFP, ultrasound, and others.
- ○ Investigate childbirth classes.

- ○ Does your boss know you're pregnant?
- ○ Start looking at maternity clothes, as your belly can grow overnight.

Fifth Month
Mother
- Still feeling good.
- Belly begins to bulge more, uterus is to your navel.
- Kidneys work harder in pregnancy.
- May notice baby movements, but not regularly (more likely if this is not your first baby).

Baby
- Teeth buds are forming.
- Baby girls will begin having primitive eggs in the ovaries.
- Gender usually distinguishable via ultrasound.
- Body covered with lanugo.
- May startle to loud, external noise.
- The weight is now up to 10 ounces (283 grams) and the baby measures about 25 cm total length, about 9.8 inches.

Things to do this month:
- ○ Sign up for childbirth classes.
- ○ Begin meeting with doulas.
- ○ Finalize plans for where you will give birth and pre-register.
- ○ Get a supply list from your midwife for a home birth.

Sixth Month
Mother
- May need to eat smaller, more frequent meals.
- Feel baby often, though may be not regularly.
- May begin to notice Braxton-Hicks contractions.

- Toward the end of this month, you may begin to feel more uncomfortable.

Baby
- Brown fat is being laid down to insulate the baby at birth.
- Eyebrows are forming.
- Practices breathing for preparation for outside life.
- Weighs in at 1 lb 5 ounces (595 grams) and 30 cm or 11.8 inches total length.
- Has chance of survival, though small, if born now.

Things to do this month:
- ○ Finish interviewing and select a doula.
- ○ Interview pediatrician.
- ○ Begin work on birth plan.
- ○ Consider diapering options.
- ○ Take additional classes, like breastfeeding and infant safety.
- ○ Register for baby registries.

THIRD TRIMESTER

Seventh Month
Mother
- Feels baby often, sometimes in a predictable pattern.
- Belly is really growing.
- Waddling a bit more as relaxin prepares body for birth.
- Prenatal appointments may be every other week now.

Baby
- May be head down in preparation for birth.
- Baby boy's testes begin descending.

- Has sleep/wake cycles.
- Your baby is about 13.8 inches long (35 cm) and weighs about 2 pounds 4 ounces (1 kilogram)!
- Better chance of survival if born now.

Things to do this month:
- ○ Consider testing like gestational diabetes screening.
- ○ Practice relaxation and other childbirth class exercises.
- ○ Make a list of what to pack for the place of birth.
- ○ Take another tour to refresh your memory.
- ○ Hire a pediatrician.

Eighth Month
Mother
- You may grow fatigued easily; nap when you can.
- Heartburn may grow worse.
- Ligaments in the hips and pelvic area are stretching in preparation for birth.
- Urination increases; always know where the closest bathroom is located.

Baby
- Nails grow and extend to tips of fingers and toes.
- Irises contract and dilate in response to light.
- Lung maturity is still continuing daily.
- Average weight of 3 pounds 11 ounces (1.7 kilograms), and measurements to 40 cm or 15.8 inches!

Things to do this month:
- ○ If you're planning a home birth, order your birth kit early this month.
- ○ Finalize birth plan, share with practitioner.
- ○ Prepare at work for your maternity leave.

- ○ Attend a blessingway or baby shower.
- ○ Have your car seat ready!
- ○ Buy diapers (cloth or disposable) or order diaper service.

Ninth Month
Mother
- Your uterus is approximately 40 cm from your pubic bone.
- Prenatal appointments may be weekly until birth.
- Common late trimester symptoms may be annoying (contractions, heartburn, insomnia, fatigue).
- Breasts may leak colostrum, but not always.

Baby
- Heart pumps 300 quarts of blood a day.
- 96 percent of babies are in a head-down position.
- Bones of the skull shaped to fit through pelvis in labor.
- Lanugo is mostly gone, though you may find patches.
- Will signal the mother when labor should start.

Things to do this month:
- ○ Fetal kick counts to help pay attention to baby's health.
- ○ Double-check packed bags for missing items.
- ○ Continue to practice labor positions and relaxation.
- ○ Do a belly cast, belly photos, or other memorable event for the end of pregnancy.

Labor
Five things you can do in early labor:
- ○ Do not pay attention to contractions too soon.

- Alternative periods of rest and activity.
- Have a project to do, like baking a cake or working on a quilt.
- Finalize plans for hospital or get your birth kit ready for a home birth.
- Eat and drink to comfort.

Five things you can do in active labor:
- Be sure to relax between contractions.
- Use comfort measures as needed.
- Consider calling your doula or other support people to help.
- Decide when to go to the hospital or call your midwife.
- Time contractions every couple of hours.

Five things you can do in transition:
- Remember to take the contractions one at a time.
- Change position often.
- Have someone with you constantly.
- Use cool cloths on your face and neck.

Five things to do while pushing:
- Stay upright to allow baby to descend.
- Enjoy the breaks between contractions.
- Remember to find your groove in pushing.
- Use your voice to help you push.
- Warm compresses and massage for your perineum can help.

Five things you can do if labor is long:
- Do not pay attention too soon.
- Grab naps whenever you can, even if it's only for a few minutes.
- Eat and drink to comfort.

- See if you can call in reinforcement support, like a backup doula.
- Change scenery if possible.

Five things you can do if labor is fast:
- Hang on. Relax.
- Try side-lying positions to slow the speed.
- Have good support with you constantly.
- Try the hands-and-knees position to help ease pain.
- Use the comfort measures that work for you, like a tub.

Five things you can do for back labor:
- Try the hands-and-knees position to help ease pain.
- Apply counterpressure to lower back.
- Apply cold compress on lower back.
- Do a double hip squeeze.
- Lunge to turn a posterior baby.

Five things your partner can do:
- Remind you to use the bathroom.
- Help you change positions.
- Advocate for you during labor.
- Take care of himself (snacks, bathroom, etc.).
- Know where your birth plan is and who to call when.

Five things you can do to prevent a cesarean:
- Choose a practitioner with a low primary cesarean rate.
- Choose a place of birth that supports natural birth.
- Move around in labor.

- Get good support from qualified help.
- Be knowledgeable about the benefits/risks of medications and interventions.

Five things you should do during a cesarean:
- Make sure all of your questions are answered.
- Have a mirror placed so you can see your baby born.
- Understand the medications used to prevent pain during and after surgery.
- Have someone go to your surgery to assist you emotionally.
- Get breastfeeding support very early.

Breastfeeding

Five things to remember while nursing:
- Know how to latch your baby on.
- Understand your baby's feeding cues.
- Find a couple of good positions to nurse in.
- Know when to get help from professionals.
- Find support in your community.

Appendix C

Other Sites and Further Readings

WEB SITES

Fertility

About Infertility Guide
http://infertility.about.com

American Society for Reproductive Medicine (ASRM)
www.asrm.org

Couple to Couple League
www.ccli.org

The International Council on Infertility Information Dissemination, Inc. (INCIID)
www.inciid.org

RESOLVE: The National Infertility Association
www.resolve.org

Society for Assisted Reproductive Technology (SART)
www.sart.org

Pregnancy

About Pregnancy Guide
http://pregnancy.about.com

Birth Activist
www.birthactivist.com

Childbirth.org
www.childbirth.org

Lamaze Institute for Normal Birth
www.normalbirth.lamaze.org

Birth Policy
www.birthpolicy.org

Vaginal Birth After Cesarean (VBAC)

www.vbac.com

American Academy of Husband-Coached Childbirth (Bradley Method)

www.bradleybirth.com

American Academy of Pediatrics (AAP)

www.aap.org

American College of Nurse Midwives (ACNM)

www.midwife.org

American College of Obstetricians and Gynecologists (ACOG)

www.acog.org

Childbirth Connection

www.childbirthconnection.org

Citizens for Midwifery (CfM)

www.cfmidwifery.org

Coalition for Improving Maternity Services (CIMS)

www.motherfriendly.org

DONA International

www.dona.org

International Cesarean Awareness Network (ICAN)

www.ican-online.org

International Childbirth Education Association (ICEA)

www.icea.org

Lamaze International
www.lamaze.org

Midwives Alliance of North America (MANA)
www.mana.org

Postpartum

Postpartum Support International (PSI)
www.postpartum.net

Depression After Delivery (DAD)
www.depressionafterdelivery.com

Fit Pregnancy
www.fitpregnancy.com

Walking Guide at About
http://walking.about.com

Breastfeeding

International Lactation Consultant Association (ILCA)
www.ilca.org

Breastfeeding Café
www.breastfeedingcafe.com

Breastfeeding Online
www.breastfeedingonline.com

La Leche League
www.lalecheleague.org

Multiples

About Parenting Multiples
http://multiples.about.com

AP Multiples
http://groups.yahoo.com/group/apmultiples

National Organization of Mothers of Twins Clubs (NOMOTC)
www.nomotc.org

Pregnancy Loss

Center for Loss in Multiple Birth (CLIMB)
www.climb-support.org

SHARE
www.nationashareoffice.com

SIDS Alliance
www.sidsalliance.org

BOOKS

Fertility

Taking Charge of Your Fertility, by Toni Weschler, MPH
The Everything Getting Pregnant Book, by Robin Elise Weiss, Certified Childbirth Educator

Pregnancy

The Official Lamaze Guide, by Judy Lothian, Ph.D., and Charlotte Devries
The Birth Partner, by Penny Simkin
The Baby Name Wizard, by Laura Wattenberg
The Birth Book, by William Sears, MD
The Pregnancy Book, by William Sears, MD, Martha Sears, RN, IBCLC
Birthing from Within, by Pam England
VBAC Companion, by Diana Korte
Blessingways: A Guide to Mother Centered Baby Showers, by Shari Maser
The Thinking Woman's Guide to a Better Birth, by Henci Goer
The Everything Pregnancy Fitness Book, by Robin Elise Weiss, Certified Childbirth Educator

Postpartum

Laughter and Tears, by Elisabeth Bing and Libby Coleman
Rebounding from Childbirth, by Lynn Madsen
This Isn't What I Expected, by Karen Kleiman and Valerie Raskin
Eat Well, Lose Weight While Breastfeeding, by Eileen Behan
Essential Exercises for the Childbearing Year, by Elizabeth Noble
The Everything Mother's First Year Book, by Robin Elise Weiss, Certified Childbirth Educator

Breastfeeding

The Nursing Mother's Companion, by Kathleen Huggins
Breastfeeding Made Simple, by Nancy Mohrbacher
Breastfeeding Café, by Barbara Behrmann
The Ultimate Breastfeeding Books of Answers, by Dr. Jack Newman and Teresa Pitman
So That's What They're For! by Janet Tomaro

Multiples

Mothering Multiples, by Karen Kerkoff Gromada, IBCLC
Expecting Twins, Triplets or Quads, by Dr. Barbara Luke
Having Twins, by Elizabeth Noble

Parenting

The No Cry Sleep Solution, by Elizabeth Pantley
The Baby Book, by Dr. William Sears
The Happiest Baby on the Block, by Harvey Karp, MD

Pregnancy Loss

Silent Sorrow, by Perry Lynn-Moffitt
Miscarriage: Women Sharing from the Heart, by Marie Allen and Shelly Marks
Trying Again: A Guide to Pregnancy After Miscarriage, Stillbirth, and Infant Loss, by Ann Douglas and John R. Sussman, MD

INDEX